T4-AJZ-137

Mental Health Care
of the Aging

Carl Eisdorfer, Ph.D., M.D., is President of the Montefiore Medical Center and Professor of Psychiatry and Neuroscience, Albert Einstein College of Medicine and Montefiore Medical Center in New York.

Donna Cohen, Ph.D., is Associate Professor of Psychiatry and Neuroscience, Albert Einstein College of Medicine and Montefiore Medical Center, and Director, Division of Aging and Geriatric Psychiatry. She is also Director of Research and Education of the Beth Abraham Hospital.

This volume was written while both authors were in the Department of Psychiatry and Behavioral Sciences, University of Washington in Seattle. Dr. Eisdorfer was professor and chairman of the department, and Dr. Cohen was an associate professor.

Mental Health Care of the Aging

A Multidisciplinary Curriculum for Professional Training

Carl Eisdorfer, Ph.D., M.D.
Donna Cohen, Ph.D.

SPRINGER PUBLISHING COMPANY
NEW YORK

Springer Publishing Company, Inc.
200 Park Avenue South
New York, New York 10003

82 83 84 85 86 / 10 9 8 7 6 5 4 3 2 1

Library of Congress Cataloging in Publication Data

Eisdorfer, Carl.
    Mental health care of the aging.

    Bibliography: p.
    Includes index.
    1. Aged—Mental health services—Study and teaching.   2. Geriatric
psychiatry—Study and teaching.   3. Aged—Services for—Study and
teaching.   I. Cohen, Donna.   II. Title. [DNLM: 1. Geriatric psychiatry—Education. WT 18 E36m]
    RC451.4.A5E38   362.2'0880565   82–5441
    ISBN 0–8261–4090–4   AACR2

Printed in the United States of America

For Isabelle . . . a vigorous, productive, involved, and giving human being, a model for all who come to know, admire, and love her.

For her eightieth birthday, September 13, 1981.

Contents

Preface

The striking and shameful inadequacies in our provision of care for the mental health problems of the aged are now a matter of public record. A number of factors, including uninformed public opinion, financial constraints, and a nihilistic belief concerning the value of mental health care for older persons have contributed to this situation. Our failure to address these problems is at least partly explained by the limited number of professionals who are educated about the factors that promote mental health as well as contribute to psychopathology in older persons. Trained mental health specialists (including but not limited to psychiatrists, psychologists, social workers, and nurses) with career commitments to the aged are needed.

Comprehensive educational programs are necessary for training mental health professionals. The goals of such programs should be to educate professionals who can not only respond to the clinical needs of the aged, but who can also facilitate the research desperately needed to improve our diagnostic and treatment strategies. To develop competent leadership in the development and delivery of mental health services to older persons is to promote the health of our older population. The latter requires that health professionals learn how to involve older persons in their own health care as well.

It has become popular to blame professionals for a lack of caring and training, and to criticize governments for poor organization, false economics, and a paucity of support services to serve as alternatives to quality medical care. However, the risk factors for cardiovascular disease and cancer, which remain our major killers and cripplers, lie squarely in the domain of individual behavior. Smoking, poor diet, lack of exercise, use of alcohol, mixtures of drugs unrelated to physician prescriptions, the reluctance to seek professional medical, psychiatric, and social health services, and an acceptance of disability as "old age" all contribute to the toll. We must be careful not to blame the patient for the disease, but we are equally at fault if we infantilize the patient or ignore the patient's own part in his or her problem. Good health care cannot be achieved purely with one-sided measures.

The financing of health care is based upon a philosophy that many of us take for granted: Physicians and other professionals in the health care system should cure. Although a cure is not always possible, increased functional capacity as an outcome of health care services is a desirable and important goal. However, even this more modest goal is not always achieved in our health care of the aged.

How much care are we willing to provide? How should we pay for it to insure the maximum effect? How can we do more to involve older persons in their own care and to help families provide care? How can we attract professionals to serve the health and mental health needs of the elderly? How can we best train them? Who should make the high-technology life and death decisions? These and a host of other questions need to be addressed, including the troublesome and haunting issue: Why, if dysfunction and death will eventually take us anyway, should we spend our money and person power just to keep people alive? The answers lie with the readers of this volume. Good health, just like good medical care, is not merely the provision of good working equipment; without a purpose for that equipment, its use is an exercise in futility. The true challenge, then, is: good health for what?

I
Objectives and Components of Training

1
Introduction

The need for a wide spectrum of health care professionals with developed expertise in providing health care to the aged is clear: The elderly are and will continue to be heavy consumers of medical care. Although they comprise 11 percent of the population at this time, they account for approximately 30 percent of the increasing national expenditures on health (Kovar, 1977; Gibson, Mueller, & Fisher,1977; Gibson & Fisher, 1978). A thorough review of health status and utilization of health care services by older persons is available elsewhere (Kovar, 1977; see also Chapters 6 through 9). However a few statistics are worth reviewing.

In 1975, an estimated $42 billion were spent on the aged (or $1,700 per person compared to $490 per person for the rest of the population). Older persons consume about 25 percent of all prescription drugs and perhaps a larger proportion of over-the-counter medication (Eisdorfer & Basen, 1979). The elderly make more office visits to physicians than younger adults, and they are admitted to general hospitals approximately two-and-a-half times more frequently than the rest of the adult population (Cantor & Mayer, 1972). Indeed, they comprise 30 percent of the adult population in hospital, medical, and surgical wards (Somers & Somers, 1967). Older persons occupy over 90 percent of the long-term care facility beds (Comptroller General's Report to Congress, 1980), and there are estimates of millions more in the community who would benefit from appropriate care. The financial reality is that nursing home care alone results in expenditures of approximately $15–16 billion a year, and the cost is growing.

3

CHALLENGE OF LONG-TERM CARE

Comprehensive long-term care is one of the most pressing and difficult of all the health care issues facing our country. Nursing home beds have increased to the point where there are now more nursing home beds in the United States than general medical and surgical hospital beds—1.2 million in contrast to one million (NCHS, 1979). It is also estimated that at least one-third of residents in nursing homes could be living elsewhere (Bell, 1973), and as many as 50 percent would like to be elsewhere (Noelker & Harel, 1978). Furthermore, the quality of care, medical and psychiatric, for the current nursing home population is questionable.

Unfortunately, dealing with the elderly, who are at increased risk for psychiatric disorder, has not been popular with mental health professionals, who may regard the aged as hopeless, helpless, and unworthy of evaluation (Cyrus-Lutz & Gaitz, 1972; Kahana & Coe, 1969; Kosberg & Cohen, 1972; Miller, Lowenstein, & Winston, 1976; Wolk & Wolk, 1971).

In view of the data, which indicate that both the number of older persons and the cost of long-term care have continued to increase (Brody, Poulshock, & Masciocchi, 1978; Eisdorfer, Cohen, & Preston, 1981), it is also unfortunate that governmental fiscal policies have done little to support either the functional evaluation of older persons for care at home or for alternative living arrangements. For example, Medicaid's long-term care support goes to institutional care rather than to community-based health services (Comptroller General's Report, 1980). Many policy and fiscal changes will be necessary to improve the state of institutional care.

PREVALENCE OF PSYCHOPATHOLOGY

Older persons are reluctant to identify their problems as psychiatric disorders, and this makes assessing the true prevalence of psychopathology in the elderly difficult. The estimated prevalence of psychiatric disorders among the elderly living in the community is reported to range from 20 to 45 percent (Bremer, 1951; Busse,

Dovenmuehle, & Brown, 1960; Busse & Pfeiffer, 1975; Gruenberg, 1978; Kay, 1977; Kay, Beamish, & Roth, 1964). The prevalence of psychiatric disorders in long-term care residents—who have an average of four chronic diseases upon admission—is also very high but woefully undocumented. Even more distressing is the estimate that at least 60 percent of residents in long-term care have an inaccurate or missing secondary diagnosis, most often related to psychiatric problems.

Psychiatric disorders may be associated with a particularly high rate of chronic and acute physical illness which may produce crippling disability and hospitalization (Lowenthal & Berkman, 1967). However, the utilization of psychiatric outpatient facilities by the aged is far less than that of the young (Kramer, Taube, & Redick, 1973). Estimates are that as many as 50 percent of older medical and surgical patients show some psychopathology (Busse & Pfeiffer, 1977; Schuckit, Miller, & Hahlbohm, 1975). Schuckit (1977b) reported that 22 percent of 327 older persons admitted to an acute medical or surgical ward of a VA Hospital over a one-year period met the criteria for a psychiatric disorder. The rate was even higher (30%) among the subgroup with cardiac problems. Alcohol abuse and drug-related problems are also significant mental health difficulties frequently seen among the aged (Eisdorfer & Basen, 1979; Schuckit, 1977a).

Frequently, psychiatric disorders are overlooked and not recorded among older persons, and it has been estimated that there may be at least a 30 percent rate of incorrect diagnosis of older persons, which would mean an even greater morbidity than that documented (Kidd, 1962). Mental changes may be noted, but often they are regarded as part of the aging process and believed to be irreversible. As a consequence, differential diagnosis and treatment that might alleviate impairments are either overlooked or disregarded. Extension of knowledge regarding the nature and course of psychopathology in the elderly, the development of new forms of therapeutic intervention, and training in a comprehensive geriatric psychiatry health care system offer the greatest hope for prolonging the productive life of the growing proportion of aged in the population, who are at risk for significant mental and emotional impairment.

COMPLEX NATURE OF ILLNESS IN THE AGED

Many diseases of the aged present with atypical or missing symptoms. The coexistence of multiple disorders and problems further complicates differential diagnosis, as does the pattern of multiple drug and physician use. Old diseases may mask symptoms of a new disease which, if undetected, increases frailty and deterioration needlessly (Brocklehurst, 1973; Ferguson Anderson, 1971; Rossman, 1971).

Economic, social, and personal losses are significant factors in the illness behavior of the aged. They often exacerbate the manifestations of disease. For example, individuals who outlive their spouses tend to become more isolated and vulnerable; this may in turn result in a magnification of the consequences of a disorder. Even a minor problem can lead to a hospital or nursing home admission because it is impossible or impractical to cope with the illness alone at home. The displacement into the institution may itself have traumatic sequelae. Many common illnesses are prolonged, and recovery from acute disturbances may proceed very slowly for the older patient.

TRAINING MENTAL HEALTH PROFESSIONALS
FOR THE FUTURE

Older patients with multiple disorders are exacting diagnostic and management challenges. The mental health problems of the aged are complicated by biological, psychological, and social factors associated with primary aging, as well as by the secondary consequences of aging in our society.

A major educational and training effort is justified for the professionals who will treat the patterns of illness in this high-risk population. Training for practice requires the development of an understanding of the unique features of older persons' mental health problems, their modes of presentation, and their interaction with other factors. Also included in training must be basic instruction on mental health and health care delivery and on the normal aging process in order to develop a basis for understanding the state of the individual.

The development of training programs which address the health and mental health needs of older persons is a matter of increasing importance (Akpom & Mayer, 1978; Butler, 1975; Dans & Kerr, 1979; Eisdorfer, 1981; Libow, 1976; Panneton & Wesolowski, 1979). Most, if not all, professionals concerned with the delivery of health or social services to adults will find themselves dealing with older individuals or with families caring for their impaired relatives. Traditional beliefs and stereotypes have resulted in a pattern of care which strongly emphasizes custodial institutions. Policymakers and caregivers alike frequently and erroneously assume that most older patients are "incurable" or "unmanageable," and a set of fiscal and administrative policies discriminate against the provision of good mental health care to those over 65.

In recognition of the current difficulties, a number of authors have articulated the need for specialized training in geriatric medicine in general (Akpom & Mayer, 1978; Butler, 1979; Freeman, 1971; Goldman, 1974; IOM, 1978; Kane, Solomon, Beck, Keeler, & Kane, 1980; Leaf, 1977; Libow, 1976; Poe, 1975; Reichel, 1977; Somers, 1976; Stevens, 1977; Wright, 1971), and in geriatric psychiatry and clinical psychology in particular (Blumenthal, Davie, & Morycz, 1979; Butler, 1975; Cohen, 1976; Eisdorfer, 1977; Rodstein, 1973). Older persons are a high-risk population for mental health problems, and their needs are underserved. It is estimated that 80 percent of the elderly requiring mental health care are not receiving attention, and if the present trends continue, it is projected that in 1985 that figure will reach 85 percent (Kramer et al., 1973).

In our opinion, there are a number of requisites for the training of mental health professionals. These include an overview of the processes of aging, a philosophic orientation to the care of the aged, supervised instruction in evaluation, diagnosis, and treatment, an understanding of the ecosystem of the older patient, consideration of policy and financial issues in health care delivery, and knowledge of the barriers to care for older patients and their families.

This volume provides a curriculum for training of professionals across the range of mental health and related human services. There are two major sections. Part I contains five chapters, which discuss the objectives and components of a training program and a specific curriculum outline. It focuses upon the knowledge and experience needed for quality mental health care of the aged. The curriculum includes biomedical aspects of aging, social and community services, as well as policy issues. For clinical training, the program specifically covers such topics as clinical manifestations of psychopathology, diagnosis, and treatment modalities (including biologic therapies). Also presented are descriptions of a number of clinical care sites and different ways of organizing training experiences since the organization of services is a basic element of a professional training program. It is hoped that this volume will enable instructors to incorporate segments of the curriculum into ongoing courses.

Part II of this volume is composed of four chapters, which provide an overview of the important historical, philosophical, and conceptual issues in geriatric education and training. The present small cadre of academicians trained and motivated to provide leadership in aging and geriatric psychiatry is not adequate to cope with the precarious health conditions of our aged population (IOM, 1978). Our nation needs a large corps of fully trained geriatric psychiatrists, clinical psychology gerontologists, social workers, nurses, and other professionals who can provide competent clinical leadership in mental health care delivery to older persons and who can provide models for future geriatric care.

2
Objectives and Philosophy of Training for Mental Health Care of the Aging

During the process of organizing an educational program, attention is often focused on course outlines, lectures, bibliographies, and faculty speakers, and sight is sometimes lost of the program's purpose. It is important to establish a philosophy for training professionals. Prior to organizing "the course" or "the program," the faculty should develop a series of specific objectives and goals.

The philosophy underlying our curriculum is that a training program in mental health care of the aged should provide a mechanism to help the individual integrate knowledge, research, skills, and clinical work in the care of the aging and aged. This not only includes the assignment of trainees to several clinical sites and community service programs, but also requires that they assume different levels of responsibility at each site, e.g., supervised patient care at one site and administration at another. Educating the individual to function across a number of care sites helps to develop an appreciation for integrated and comprehensive networks of mental health care.

A training program should involve intensive interaction with the community, professional schools, hospitals, and other appropriate clinical settings. Lectures, seminars, and a broad range of supervised, clinical work in different settings are important to broaden the base of experience and knowledge as well as to demonstrate the appropriate use of conceptual, therapeutic, and management strategies for the care of the aged. In addition, interdisciplinary conferences and seminar experiences can help the individual in training to relate to a range of professionals as well as to understand the importance of continuity of care for older patients and their families.

The major objectives of our curriculum are to provide comprehensive training and education in mental health care and services for the aged, to develop leadership skills in clinical care, program development, and management, and to facilitate research and teaching. Specifically, at least the following three basic objectives should be met by a clinical training program:

Objective 1. To teach competence and standards of excellence in the diagnosis, treatment, management, rehabilitation, and prevention of illness and disorders in the older patient in a range of sites including clinics, hospitals, and community and long-term care settings.

The mental health professional is often confronted by patients with more than one major health problem. Psychopathology may appear in typical ways, such as anxiety, depression, or dementia. It may take other forms, such as alcoholism, drug abuse and misuse, or it may appear as exacerbations of physical diseases such as hypertension and coronary illness, respiratory disorders, and chronic pain. Older persons also may experience functional and psychosocial losses (economic, social, personal) which require sophisticated diagnostic and management skills. Firsthand experience with patients requiring an assessment of the social, behavioral, and cultural factors contributing to physical and mental disorders is essential for the education of the clinician.

In recognition of the many variables which influence patient care, training programs should develop a knowledge base which includes fundamental concepts and issues in the field of aging as well as clinical knowledge and skills. An appreciation of these more basic issues is not only relevant for clinical activity with individual patients, but it will contribute to the professional's sense of identity as an expert clinician in the field of gerontology. Understanding the aging process is also necessary as a basis for integrating newer developments in the burgeoning discipline of geriatric mental health. This training is critical for quality clinical work in the future.

A training program should teach about the unique presentations of disease, illness, and other life problems occurring in older age groups. It should also focus upon the special needs of older persons who live at home or in other settings, emphasizing the wide range of clinical and community services necessary to enhance health, dignity, and the quality of life. Clinicians in training should have the opportunity to evaluate and intervene with the major adaptational problems and psychiatric diseases known to occur in the later years of life, e.g. multiple chronic health problems, existential sadness, dementia, depressions, and multiple medications.

The personality dynamics and coping mechanisms of older patients have a significant impact on health behavior. It is important that any training program teach the concept of behavior as the end product of a complex biopsychosocial process; this enables the professional to understand and to know how to mediate the many influences affecting successful or maladaptive behavior.

Clinicians should be taught the following skills:

1. To analyze and define those behavioral, social, physical, and cultural factors that mediate illness and disease, and to make accurate differential diagnosis of various mental health problems affecting the aged;

2. To understand the effects of medical illness on patient behavior and affect, and to appreciate the physical manifestations of psychiatric disorders;

3. To appreciate the intrapsychic as well as social and cultural factors in the evaluation of mental and emotional problems in older persons;

4. To develop clinical skills across a range of behavioral, psychodynamic, and psychopharmacologic (and other biologic) therapies;

5. To specify objectives of treatment, rehabilitation, management, and intervention programs;

6.   To design behavioral, social, and somatic strategies to obtain these objectives;

7.   To apply knowledge and skills in a variety of health care sites;

8.   To learn about sources of information and referral for patients and families in the community;

9.   To understand and appreciate the importance of practical issues in the life of the patient;

10.   To evaluate the efficacy of treatment programs.

Objective II.   To develop an understanding of a range of health and social service disciplines in the care of the aged and to develop skills at collaboration, program management, and the development and evaluation of a variety of models of care.

Opportunities to observe, work in, and assess the operations of a variety of programs are important. The elderly are not confined to one type of setting, and the clinician must learn about the range of needs of older persons, in a number of different settings, including the home, the community, the hospital, and the long-term care facility.

Skills in program development can be learned in seminars and lecture programs as can an understanding of community needs and services available to the aged. Specifically, the trainee should be taught the following:

1.   To understand the social and ecological antecedents to illness in the elderly;

2.   To identify and intervene against the preventable antecedents;

3.   To identify and/or facilitate the development of critical support mechanisms for patients in order to maximize self-esteem and independence;

4.   To develop special health-related educational and training programs for older persons to help them utilize their external support systems and make them educated advocates of quality care;

5. To facilitate the use of available community services and to help develop better services to meet the future needs of the aged;

6. To reduce barriers of an historic, economic, sexual, racial, or age-related nature among health care professionals and staff in order to provide optimal care for older persons.

Objective III. To develop a knowledge of research activity and scholarship concurrently with clinical acumen in the interest of improving the quality of health care intervention, strategies, assessment tools, and services based upon empirical data.

Clinical excellence requires that the individual develop and maintain an awareness of ongoing research and understand the importance of incorporating new information to improve care. Research opportunities should be identified in several areas, including basic and clinical research, health policy, health services, and evaluation of community needs. Responsible clinicians and agencies can play an important role in research and problem solving oriented to improving patient care. Improved data collection, the use of more explicit records, and an understanding of the value of such information can be of direct benefit, not only to researchers, but also to the patients and staff involved. The trainee should be taught state-of-the-art techniques of care as well as an appreciation of the attitude that "there may be a better way." Specifically, the program should provide opportunities for trainees in the following:

1. To learn about ongoing research and to develop an appreciation for the need to continue one's education in professional practice;

2. To participate in such clinical research as is appropriate to expand a conceptual framework and to develop an ability to understand empirical methods for clinical decision making;

3. To develop and understand how to conduct programs of community support and/or intervention.

In summary, training should aim to achieve a set of objectives based on a philosophy. For our curriculum, we propose the following: (1) The promotion of clinical excellence and the development of leadership potential in conjunction with the development of clinical, research, training, and administrative capabilities; (2) investing trainees with a knowledge of the aging process; (3) training to provide quality clinical care; (4) integration of mental health delivery within the existing network of aging services in the community; (5) understanding the limitations for service delivery which currently exist; and (6) the development of new alternatives to meet the emerging needs of the impaired aged.

3

A Program for the Training of Mental Health Professionals in Aging

A training program for specialized practice in the mental health of the aged should have the following major components: Clinical experience in inpatient and outpatient psychiatric settings, as well as community consultation; a core group of seminars, including concepts of normal aging, principles of clinical diagnosis and management, and health policy and health management; and clinical research training. The program emphasizes specialty training and the acquisition of experience in an interdisciplinary health team at different sites in the mental health care system.

This is an advanced training program that should be considered an addition to the basic professional education of the individual. Thus, psychiatrists should have completed an internship and at least two years of general residency training; clinical psychologists should have completed their Ph.D. degree requirements, including an internship; social workers and nurses should be at the Master's level or with appropriate clinical and educational backgrounds.

The use of this curriculum, however, is not restricted to the training of advanced specialists. Preprofessional and professional training goals may also be served by employing the lecture and seminar material that follows. Our purpose in presenting the advanced training program with its tracks as the primary model is to organize the range of information, clinical skills, and interactions which geriatric mental health professionals must master. Individual training sites and faculty may employ all, or only elements, of the material here for the purposes of specific programs. The gamut of issues affecting the mental and emotional well-being of older persons should be widely taught, and an understanding of the range of manifestations of psychopathology and maladaptation is an essential for all clinicians. Finally, a goal for all programs, at whatever level, should be to instill in professionals a recognition of the value of careful evalution of all older patients and of the great potential for successful treatment outcome in many instances.

A two-year training program with a common core, but with unique elements for each specialty area, is optimal for the development of competence in the clinical care of the aged. The first year includes a range of supervised clinical experiences, while the second year provides three optional opportunities for trainees. Option A is an Advanced Clinician Track in geriatric mental health. Option B is a Mental Health Policy and Management Track. Option C is a Clinical Research and Teaching (or Academic) track. In the second year, at least 50 percent of an individual's time continues to be spent in supervised clinical training, while the remaining time is organized according to individual interests within the framework of the available options.

The program should be designed to develop the following skills, attitudes, and knowledge during clinical training.

Skills

1. Differential Diagnosis of Psychiatric Disorders in the Aged
2. Functional Assessment of the Aged Patient
3. Interdisciplinary Team Cooperation
4. Psychodiagnostics
5. Individual and Group Treatment, Rehabilitation, and Management
6. Pharmacologic Management and Treatment
7. Behavioral Therapies
8. Dealing with Death and Dying
9. Family Care
10. Management of Comprehensive Care

11.   Utilization of Community Resources
12.   Exercise of Clinical Inference Using a Data Base
13.   Application of Scientific Methods to Understanding Problems of the Aging and the Aged
14.   Consultation with Other Physicians
15.   Dealing with Institutional Management

Attitudes

1.   Development of a Positive, Nonprejudicial Approach to Elderly Patients and Their Families
2.   Development of an Understanding of Patient–Clinician Interaction
3.   Development of a Behavioral-Ecological Approach to Patient Illness and Care
4.   Development of a Humane and Rational Approach to the Care of the Dying Patient and toward the Family and Staff Involved in Patient Care
5.   Development of an Understanding of the Stresses, Adjustments, and Adaptations of the Aging and Aged

Knowledge

1.   Understanding of Health and Disease in the Aged (Primary and Secondary Aging)
2.   Normal Variation in Behavior with Advancing Age
3.   Impact of the Environment on the Individual
4.   Illness Behavior in the Aged
5.   The Etiology of Emotional Disorders in the Aged
6.   Differential Diagnosis and Treatment of Cognitive Dysfunction in the Aged
7.   Differential Diagnosis and Treatment of Depression
8.   Understanding of Paranoid and Schizophrenic States
9.   Understanding of Anxiety States
10.   Drug Abuse and Alcoholism

11.   Patient Treatment and Management: Orchestrating Maximum Function and Minimum Dependence at a Reasonable Cost

12.   Psychotherapeutic Strategies (Individual and Group)

13.   Behavioral Treatment Strategies

14.   Understanding of Family Relationships and Family Therapy

15.   Psychopharmacology

16.   Prevention of Illness and Disease

17.   Management of the Dying Patient

18.   Health Strategies and Policies

CURRICULUM PLANS

The two-year fellowship program stresses a multidisciplinary approach to mental health care. Although the various clinical training sites emphasize the unique aspects of each specialty, patient care conferences, seminars, and lectures in aging and geriatric mental health are broad-ranging in approach.

In the first year, individuals rotate through clinical services and participate in seminars and lectures. In the second year they have the option of concentrating on advanced clinical training or of spending up to 50 percent of their time either in clinical research and academic studies or in mental health and health policy and management studies.

CLINICAL TRAINING SITES AND
THEIR SKILLS OPPORTUNITIES

There are at least six areas in which individuals should be trained:

1.   Acute Inpatient Care

2.   Chronic Inpatient Care

3.   Subacute Care

4. Outpatient Care
5. Family Care
6. Consultation Services

Acute Inpatient Care

The skills that can be developed in acute inpatient care sites include:

1. Differential diagnosis of cognitive and emotional problems, with consultation from the Department of Medicine
2. Assessment of acute psychiatric problems
3. Drug evaluation therapy
4. Family crisis intervention
5. Psychological evaluation
6. Discharge planning and follow-up
7. Research

Chronic Inpatient Care

One goal of the training faculty should be to provide access to an inpatient unit designed specifically for the care of cognitively impaired aged persons with primary neuronal degeneration of the Alzheimer's type who require long-term institutionalization. Such a unit provides a structured, stimulating, and pleasant environment to assist patients in adapting and coping with cognitive and emotional changes without psychopharmacologic agents. It also provides a controlled environment for clinical research by which we can improve our data base to characterize, manage, and rehabilitate persons with the Alzheimer's type of dementia. Techniques include contingency therapies, family involvement, and family therapy interaction. Training on an inpatient chronic care unit should encompass:

1. Differential diagnosis of primary neuronal degeneration of the Alzheimer's Type

2. Behavioral management techniques using minimum psychoactive medications

3. Staff management

4. Evaluations of impact of the disease upon nuclear family groups

5. Assessment of psychological, neurological, cardiovascular, and metabolic anomalies that may have impact on the progression of the disease

6. Clinical research in a controlled clinical care environment

Subacute Care

Subacute care is intermediate between long-term institutional care and the acute hospital bed. The Subacute Care Unit can serve as the focus for an overall program in geriatric medicine, encompassing a geriatric outpatient clinic, day hospital program, nursing home consultation, and research programs in clinical and health services. A wide range of training is possible in the Subacute Care Unit:

1. Evaluation and consultation by an interdisciplinary team of an internist, psychiatrist, nurse, social worker, and psychologist. Evaluations may allow direct disposition to home, acute medical facility, or nursing homes. The Subacute Care Unit provides a focus for instruction in diagnostic procedures and in-depth evaluation of social or long-term support needs.

2. Discharge planning which facilitates community placement. Discharge of elderly patients, especially from acute medical facilities, is often delayed long after hospitalization is no longer necessary. The patient's social, economic and environmental problems are very important in appropriate disposition.

3. Care of subacute and recurrent problems with short hospital stays. The purpose of the short-stay admission is to avoid long and expensive hospitalization on an acute ward or in a nursing home. Short-stay, repeated admissions with discharge to patients' own homes or nursing home facilities will provide trainees with opportunities to closely control and adjust, if necessary, patients' diet, activity, and medications.

4.   Care of the terminally ill with intermittent hospitalization. The unit can interact with community-based health programs so that planned hospitalization is designed to alleviate pain and promote dignity in the dying process.

5.   Interdisciplinary education and training to develop an understanding of critical support systems within and without the health care system.

6.   Multidisciplinary research opportunities to combine clinical and research experiences relevant to those training for an academic career.

Outpatient Sites

Opportunities for learning in the outpatient setting include:

1.   Multidisciplinary assessment of patients and their families
2.   Assessment of multiple problems
3.   Family as well as individual counseling and therapy
4.   Evaluation of barriers to home health care
5.   Assessment of level of care
6.   Death and dying
7.   Research

Family Care

A Geriatric and Family Services Clinic is a specialized outpatient program designed to provide direct medical and psychiatric services to the elderly as well as information and counseling for families of the elderly. Specific skills and opportunities include:

1.   Multidisciplinary team assessment of patients and their families by a team of psychiatrist, internist, nurse, and social worker

2.   Family counseling and therapy

3.   Home visits

4.   Evaluation of barriers (including architectural barriers) to home health maintenance

5.   Assessment of level of care

6.   Management of the dying patient

7.   Research opportunities

Consultation Services

Trainees should do consultation in a number of sites, in community-based clinics as well as for geriatric day health, geriatric home health, and other hospital services. Special opportunities include:

1.   Diagnosis, management, treatment, and rehabilitation of psychiatric problems in the elderly in nursing homes and the community

2.   Consultation with other professionals in the community and hospital environment

3.   Evaluation of the impact of living arrangements and the psychosocial environment on illness and disease

4.   Knowledge of community care system for the aged

PROGRAM OF STUDY: ROTATION FOR CLINICAL PRACTICE SPECIALTY AND ACADEMICALLY ORIENTED PROFESSIONALS

Year 1

The first year is devoted to intensive clinical training with rotations designed to teach the elements of continuity of care and to emphasize a broad-based approach to patient care. In the first year trainees spend: four months (100% time) in an inpatient acute care unit; four months (50% time) in a Chronic Care Unit and a Subacute Care Unit (50% time); and four months in an Outpatient Service (50% time) and a consultation site (50% time). Tables 3.1–3.3 present sample weekly schedules for the Year 1 rotations.

TABLE 3.1

Sample Weekly Schedule for Year 1 Geriatric Mental Health Professionals (50
Percent Acute Inpatient and 50 Percent Outpatient Care)

Monday	Tuesday	Wednesday	Thursday	Friday
Unit Work, Rounds, and Patient Care: 0800-1130 Hrs.	Unit Work, Rounds, and Patient Care: 0800-1000 Hrs.	Research on Inpatient Unit: 0800-1300 Hrs.		Research on Inpatient Unit: 0800-1130 Hrs.
	Weekly Teaching Rounds: 1000-1130 Hrs.			
Attending Teaching Rounds: 1400-1530 Hrs.	Attending Teaching Rounds: 1400-1530 Hrs.	Unit Work and Patient Care: 1500-1800 Hrs.	Attending Teaching Rounds: 1400-1530 Hrs.	
Unit Work, Rounds, Patient Care, and Consultation: 1530-1800 Hrs.	Independent Study Time with Supervisor: 1600-1800 Hrs.		Unit Work, Rounds, and Patient Care: 1530-1800 Hrs.	Unit Work, Rounds, and Patient Care: 1600-1800 Hrs.

23

TABLE 3.2

Sample Weekly Schedule for Year 1 Geriatric Mental Health Professionals (50 Percent Chronic Inpatient and 50 Percent Subacute Care)

Monday	Tuesday	Wednesday	Thursday	Friday
Subacute Unit Work, Rounds, and Patient Care: 0800–1200 Hrs.	Subacute Unit Work, Rounds, and Patient Care: 0800–1000 Hrs.	Chronic Inpatient Unit Work, Rounds, and Patient Care: 0800–1200 Hrs.	Didactic: 0800–1200 Hrs.	Chronic Inpatient Unit Work, Rounds, and Patient Care: 0800–1200 Hrs.
	Weekly Teaching Rounds: 1000–1130 Hrs.			
Bimonthly Behavioral Sciences Seminar: 1200–1300 Hrs.	Fellows Weekly Clinical Care Conference: 1200–1330 Hrs.			
Subacute Teaching Rounds: 1330–1500 Hrs.	Supervisory Time: 1400–1530 Hrs.	Chronic Inpatient Teaching Rounds: 1300–1430 Hrs.	Research Time: 1400–1800 Hrs.	Chronic Inpatient Teaching Rounds: 1300–1430 Hrs.
Subacute Unit Work, Rounds, and Patient Care: 1600–1800 Hrs.	Subacute Unit Work, Rounds, and Patient Care: 1600–1800 Hrs.	Aging Seminar: 1600–1800 Hrs.		Chronic Inpatient Unit Work, Rounds, and Patient Care: 1500–1800 Hrs.

TABLE 3.3
Sample Weekly Schedule for Year 1 Geriatric Mental Health Professionals (50 Percent Outpatient and 50 Percent Consultation)

Monday	Tuesday	Wednesday	Thursday	Friday
Outpatient Clinic: 0800-1200 Hrs.	Outpatient Clinic: 0800-1000 Hrs.	Outpatient Clinic: 0800-1130 Hrs.	Didactic: 0800-1200 Hrs.	Outpatient Clinic: 0800-1200 Hrs.
	Weekly Rounds: 1030-1200 Hrs.			
Bimonthly Behavioral Science Seminar: 1200-1300 Hrs.				
Consultation Site: 1300-1800 Hrs.	Fellows Weekly Clinical Care Conference: 1200-1330 Hrs.	Consultation Site: 1230-1530 Hrs.	Attending Weekly Teaching Rounds: 1330-1500 Hrs.	Consultation Site: 1300-1800 Hrs.
	Supervisory Time: 1330-1500 Hrs.			
	Home Visits: 1500-1800 Hrs.	Aging Seminar: 1600-1800 Hrs.		

Year 2

Second year trainees move into either an Advanced Clinician track, a Mental Health Policy and Management track, or a Clinical Research track. Individuals oriented toward academic careers may choose among slightly modified versions of these three tracks.

The Advanced Clinician track consists of twelve months of consultation in hospital and community sites. The Mental Health Policy and Management track is divided into two six month sections. The first six months consist of consultation in hospital and community sites (50% time) and management training (50% time). The last six months emphasize a management practicum in which trainees are placed in a supervisory position at a particular site. The Clinical Research track consists of twelve months of consultation in hospital and community sites with half the time designated for clinical research and training.

For academically oriented individuals the Advanced Clinician track consists of twelve months of consultation in hospital and community sites with 25 to 50 percent time devoted to clinical research and training. The Mental Health Policy and Management track consists of twelve months of consultation in hospital and community sites (50% time), management training (25% time), and health policy research (25% time). The Clinical Research track consists of twelve months of consultation in community and hospital sites with 50 to 100 percent of time devoted to clinical research.

CLASSROOM AND CONFERENCE TRAINING

A variety of seminars, conferences, and lectures should be included in the program.

1. First Year Orientation Seminar: When individuals begin training, they should attend orientation seminars following the sample outline in Table 3.4.
2. Teaching Conferences: All trainees should attend teaching conferences which are part of the weekly program.

3. Attending Teaching Rounds: These teaching rounds are conducted daily by attending geriatric clinicians in the inpatient and subacute settings and weekly or biweekly in the outpatient and consultation settings. All new and/or problem cases are to be discussed; discussions should involve a multidisciplinary staff.

4. Lecture Seminars: The first year lecture seminar for trainees meets weekly and covers the curriculum presented in Table 3.5. The second year is in two phases: Phase I is a weekly meeting for all trainees covering the topics in Table 3.6; Phase II (the last six months) is a period of independent reading and supervised study.

5. Aging and Geriatric Psychiatry Seminars: The first-year seminars meet weekly and cover topics in the three major areas presented in Table 3.7: Biomedical and biobehavioral issues, social and behavioral issues, management and human services issues. Starting with the second half of Year 1, seminars alternate with a journal club, devoted to analysis of important articles, which continues into the second year.

6. Patient Care Conferences: The trainees are responsible for planning and coordinating a weekly clinical care conference. Relevant topics in relation to patient problems are presented and discussed.

TABLE 3.4

Sample Orientation First Year Seminar for Training Program on Aging for Mental Health Professionals

I.   Introduction and Structure of the Training Program

II. Overview of Aging

     A. Demographic Changes

     B. Health Characteristics of the Aged

     C. The Aged Patient and Mental Health Care

     D. Barriers to Care

     E. Advances in Clinical Care

     F. Special Problems in Patient Management

III. Comprehensive Long-Term Care

IV. Aging Research: A Review and Critique

     A. Types of Research

     B. Theories of Aging

     C. Issue of Deficits

     D. Normal Aging

     E. Psychopathology

     F. Special Problems of Aging Research

V.   Clinical Issues in the Care of the Aged

     A. Principles of Patient Care

     B. Hospital Care of the Aged

     C. Care of the Aged in the Community

     D. Treatment and Rehabilitation of the Older Patient

     E. Challenge of Geriatrics

VI. Needs of the Elderly

     A. General, Income, Employment, Housing

     B. Education, Transportation, Legal Services

     C. Physical Health, Mental Health

VII. The Aging Network

TABLE 3.5
Curriculum for the First Year Lectures

I.   Biologic Aspects of Aging

     A.   Theories of Aging

     B.   Genetics of Aging

     C.   Molecular Aging

     D.   Cellular Aging

     E.   Physiologic Functioning and Decline

     F.   Central Nervous System Changes

          1.   Neuropathology
          2.   Psychophysiology
          3.   Neuroendocrine Changes
          4.   Immunologic Alterations
          5.   Sensory Changes
          6.   Sleep Physiology

II. Psychosocial Aspects of Aging

     A.   Young Adulthood

     B.   Sex Differences During Adult Development and Aging

     C.   Families and Singles

     D.   Work, Retirement, and Leisure

     E.   Marriage and the Family

     F.   Family Changes

     G.   Middle Age

     H.   Attitudes

     I.   Old Age: Young-Old versus Old-Old

III. Other Ways of Growing Old: Cultural Differences

IV. Psychological Changes During Adult Development and Aging

     A.   Personality During Adult Development and Aging

     B.   Sensorimotor Alterations

     C.   Attention

     D.   Learning   *continued*

29

TABLE 3.5 (continued)

IV. Psychological Changes During Adult Development and Aging (continued)

    E. Memory

    F. Higher Cognitive Functioning

    G. Creativity

    H. Definition of Competence

V. Sexuality and Aging

    A. Changing Sexuality

    B. The Older Man

    C. The Older Woman

VI. The Impact of the Environment on the Aged

    A. How the Elderly Live

        1. Life Style and Location
        2. Life Space and Social Support
        3. Housing and the Urban Aged
        4. Housing and the Rural Aged
        5. Family and Social Relationships

    B. How the Elderly Negotiate the Environment

    C. Research Theory and Methodology

    D. Architectural Barriers to Health

VII. Psychopathology

    A. Dementing Disorders

    B. Depressive Disorders

    C. Paranoia and Schizophrenia

    D. Anxiety Disorders

    E. Alcohol-Related Disorders

    F. Drug Use and Abuse

    G. Sleep Disorders

    H. Neurosis and Personality Disorders

    I. Sexual Dysfunction *continued*

TABLE 3.5 (continued)

VIII. Treatment and Management

    A. Psychopharmacology

    B. Psychotherapy

    C. Behavioral Management

    D. Family Intervention

IX. Evaluation and Assessment

    A. Assessment of Psychopathology

    B. Assessment of Cognitive Dysfunction

    C. Assessment of Depression

    D. Assessment of Anxiety, Paranoia

    E. Assessment of Community Adjustment

    F. Assessment of Family and Social Support Systems

X. Long-Term Care

    A. Nursing Homes

    B. Alternatives to Institutionalization

XI. Death and Dying

    A. The Process of Dying

    B. Principles of Patient Care

31

TABLE 3.6
Curriculum for Second Year Lectures

I. Health Care Policy Issues

A. Medical Care

B. Home Care

C. Mental Health Care

D. Community Services

E. Nutrition Services

F. Housing Services

G. Institutional Care

H. Reimbursement for Services

I. Transportation and Communication Services

J. Legislated Social Services

K. Social Security

L. Medicare

M. Comprehensive Services

N. Towards a Data-based Psychiatry

O. Ethics of Geriatric Care

P. Can We Afford Health Care for the Aged

II. Elective Study

A. Track A--Advanced Clinical

B. Track B--Clinical Research

C. Track C--Management

TABLE 3.7
Topics for First Year Seminars

I.   BIOMEDICAL AND BIOBEHAVIORAL ISSUES

    A. Decline in immunocompetence with aging and its
        implications.

    B. Variations in aging process and in disease patterns
        among the aged of different ethnic and cultural groups
        as well as between the sexes.

    C. Effective diagnosis and treatment of the cognitive
        diseases.

    D. Criteria for healthy and successful aging.

    E. Death and Dying.

II. SOCIAL AND BEHAVIORAL ISSUES

    A. Life cycle crisis and adjustment

    B. Work and social roles for older people

    C. Socioeconomic costs of the aging society

    D. Family structure and patterns of aging.

    E. Middle age--the transition to old age

    F. Personality and aging

    G. Cognitive enhancement

    H. Environments for the elderly

III. MANAGEMENT AND HUMAN SERVICES

    A. Integrated services for the elderly

    B. Self-care and preventive medicine

    C. Living arrangements for the elderly

    D. The family as a social service delivery system

    E. The environment for long-term care

    F. Health care costs in aging

    G. Training in Geriatrics and Gerontology

    H. Research and training evaluation

4
A Curriculum Outline on Mental Health and Aging

The outline that follows identifies important areas of knowledge for the training of mental health professionals in the field of aging. Since the outline itself is long and detailed, an overview of the issues in each of the five major content areas is presented below.

I.   Normal Aging   p. 36
     A.   An Introduction to the Processes of Aging
     B.   Concepts and Measurement of Changes with Age
     C.   Biological Theories of Aging
     D.   Psychological Theories of Aging
     E.   Psychosocial Theories of Aging
     F.   An Integrated Approach to Understand Changes in Older Persons
     G.   Social Change for the Aging and Aged
II. Assessment and Diagnosis of Psychopathology   p. 38
     A.   Factors in Diagnosis
     B.   Interviewing the Older Patient
     C.   Behavioral Assessment of Psychopathology
     D.   Assessment of Cognitive Dysfunction
     E.   Impact of Environment on Behavior
III. Psychopathology: Manifestations and Management   p. 43
     A.   DSM-III and the Aged Patient
     B.   Dementing Illness
     C.   Depression
     D.   Anxiety Disorders
     E.   Paranoid Disorders

A CONTENT OUTLINE ON THE
PSYCHOPATHOLOGY OF AGING

I.   Normal Aging
A.   An Introduction to the Processes of Aging
   1.   Age: A process with antecedents
      a.   Primary and secondary aging
      b.   The young-old and the old-old
      c.   Increasing frailty of older persons
      d.   Compensatory processes (losses and gains)
      e.   Experience vs. deficit
   2.   Individual differences

B. Concepts and Measurement of Changes with Age
    1. Deficit or change?
        a. Descriptive models of time-related changes
        b. Disease models (aging vs. disease)
        c. Risk factor models
        d. Adaptational models
    2. Issues in the measurement of change
        a. Measures and their meaning
        b. When do biological changes predict functional
            capacity?
        c. Cohort differences
        d. Time of measurement differences
        e. Testwise-ness of subjects
        f. Motivation of subjects
        g. Age-appropriate measures
    3. Research designs
        a. Cross-sectional and longitudinal methods
        b. Sequential strategies
        c. Change in subject population with age
        d. Change in populations and sampling
    4. Modeling change over time
    5. Simulation of developmental changes
    6. Cross-cultural comparisons
    7. Structural designs
        a. Causal relationships
        b. Use of structural models
C. Biological Theories of Aging
    1. Genetic theories
    2. Nongenetic cellular theories
    3. Immunological theories
    4. Endocrine theories
    5. Free radical theory
    6. Genetic vs. stochastic theories

        7. Time vs. trauma
- D. Psychological Theories of Aging
  1. Objectives of psychological theories
     a. Description
     b. Explanation
  2. Plasticity of behavior
  3. Psychodynamic theory
  4. Theories of cognitive change
  5. Theories of personality change
  6. Biobehavioral approaches
- E. Psychosocial Theories of Aging
  1. Concomitant theory
  2. Impact of the environment on aging and behavior
  3. Impact of social structures on aging
  4. Cultural factors: Other ways of growing old
- F. An Integrated Approach to Understand Changes in Older Persons
  1. Ageism
  2. Stress, disease, and aging
  3. Competence and aging
  4. Functional age
- G. Social Change for the Aging and Aged
  1. The politics of developing and implementing policy
  2. Income distribution
  3. Distribution of health care resources
  4. Lifelong education

II. Assessment and Diagnosis of Psychopathology
- A. Factors in Diagnosis
  1. The aging patient
     a. Adaptive style of patient
        (1) Health problems and functional capacity
        (2) Support systems
        (3) Living situation
        (4) Economics

(5) Recent life events
(6) History
(7) Disease vs. Illness
  b. Patient beliefs and attitudes
  c. Family beliefs and attitudes
2. Diagnostic approaches
  a. Patient interviews
  b. Family interviews
  c. Data from other observers
  d. Psychological tests
  e. Functional assessment
  f. Criteria for diagnosis
3. Management
  a. Accurate diagnosis
  b. Multiple problems
  c. Family and social support systems
  d. Aging network in the community
B. Interviewing the Older Patient
1. Concerns of older person about implications of interview
2. Motivation for interview (older person or "surrogate parent")
3. Attention or communication problems of patient
4. Focus on recent or remote past
5. Physical and practical issues vs. psychological issues
6. Examiner anxiety
7. Touching the patient
8. Use of appropriate tests, e.g., mental status exam
9. Return appointments
10. Depth of interview
11. Setting of interview
C. Behavioral Assessment of Psychopathology
1. Areas of focus

    a. Affect
- (1) Depression
- (2) Anxiety
- (3) Paranoid behavior

    b. Cognition
- (1) Attention
- (2) Learning
- (3) Memory
- (4) Focal cognitive skills

    c. Communication skills
- (1) Language
- (2) Sensory impairments
- (3) Nonverbal communication

    d. Control behavior
- (1) Speed
- (2) Arousal

    e. Social intelligence

    f. Coping with stress

2. Conceptual and practical issues in assessment
3. Psychiatric rating scales for psychopathology
   a. Depression
   b. Anxiety
   c. Multiple psychopathology
   d. Mental status
4. Self-rating scales for psychopathology
   a. Personality inventories
   b. Depression
   c. Anxiety
   d. Mood
   e. Screening examination
5. Nurse and psychiatric aide rating scales
   a. Geriatric Rating Scale (GRS)

      b. Physical and Mental Impairment-of-function Evaluation (PAMIE)

      c. Nurses' Observation Scale for Inpatient Evaluation (NOSIE)

      d. Ward Behavior Inventory (WBI)

      e. Stockton Rating Scale (SRS)

  6. Community adjustment

      a. Standards for measurement of adjustment in the aged

      b. Adjustment rating scale

      c. Affective rating scale

  7. Cognitive performance

      a. Mental status evaluation

      b. Psychometric tests

      c. Neuropsychological tests

D. Assessment of Cognitive Dysfunction

  1. Cognitive functioning during aging and human development

      a. Effects of primary aging

      b. Effects of secondary aging

  2. A perspective on assessment

      a. Psychometric instruments

      b. Neuropsychological instruments

      c. Mental status evaluations

  3. Areas of cognitive dysfunction

  4. Goals of clinical cognitive evaluation

      a. Assess strengths and deficits

      b. Improved differential diagnosis

      c. Provide baseline to assess change

      d. Provide basis for management

  5. Language evaluation

  6. Cognitive evaluation battery

a. Attention
b. Memory
c. Focal cognitive skills
d. Clinical mental status
7. Practical applications
8. Testing the cognitively impaired aged
   a. Mild impairment
   b. Moderate impairment
   c. Severe impairment
   d. Severity vs. duration of illness
   e. Course of illness
E. Impact of Environment on Behavior
   1. Multiple losses and impact on behavior
      a. Sensory
      b. Physiological
      c. Physical mobility
      d. Psychosocial changes
   2. Person–environment relations
      a. Environmental congruence
         (1) Person (needs and preferences)
         (2) Environmental press (product demands or "press")
         (3) Adaptation/maladaptation
      b. Environment docility
         (1) Competence of individual
         (2) Potential of environment to activate behavior
      c. Measurement of person–environment relations
         (1) Needs and preferences of individual
         (2) Competence of individual
         (3) Physical health of individual
         (4) Physical environmental demands, e.g., complexity
         (5) Social environment, e.g., social network, activities

III. Psychopathology: Manifestations and Management
    A.   DSM-III and the Aged Patient
        1.   Overview and critique of DSM-III
            a.   Dementing disorders
            b.   Depressive disorders
            c.   Schizophrenia
            d.   Anxiety disorders
            e.   Other categories
        2.   Need for functional assessment
    B.   Dementing Illness
        1.   Facts and figures
            a.   Causes of brain failure
            b.   Epidemiology
            c.   Reversible dementias
            d.   Nonreversible dementias
        2.   Nature and course of nonreversible dementing illness
            a.   Primary neuronal degeneration of the Alzheimer type
                (1)   Etiology
                (2)   Brain changes
            b.   Multi-infarct dementia
                (1)   Etiology
                (2)   Brain changes
            c.   Manifestation
                (1)   Behavior
                (2)   Brain
                (3)   Family and social support system
            d.   Course of illness
        3.   Clinical tests and diagnostic procedures
            a.   Physical exam
            b.   Neurologic exam
            c.   Psychiatric exam
            d.   Psychological exam
            e.   Laboratory tests

      f.   Drug history
      g. Psychosocial history
      h. Diagnostic criteria
4. Management
      a. Maintenance of physical health
      b. Treatment of accompanying symptoms
      c. Pharmacotherapy
      d. Behavioral management
      e. Cognitive enhancement
      f.   Family support and therapy
      g. Physical activity
      h. Environmental modifications
5. Stages of the dementing process in the patient
6. Effect of dementing illness on caregiver
      a. Caregivers
          (1) Family
          (2) Social support system
      b. Coping with stress
          (1) Physical illness
          (2) Psychiatric illness
          (3) Maladjustment
7. Phases in the family reaction to dementing illness
      a. Developing awareness
          (1) Disruption . . . "something is seriously wrong"
          (2) Evaluation . . . hypothesis concerning the cause of the disruption
          (3) Reaction . . . reaction to the perceived cause
      b. Questioning
          (1) Initial belief not sufficient to account for magnitude of change
          (2) Significant event
          (3) Search for professional help

    c. Reaction to medical diagnosis

    d. Search for community resources . . . where can we get assistance?

    e. Reorganization

        (1) Altered role relationships

        (2) Bonding and new intimacy

        (3) Spouse or patient as dependent

        (4) Crisis around institutionalization

        (5) Rejection

        (6) Coping/adaptation/maladaptation

    f. Process issues

        (1) Preparation for longer-term care

        (2) Psychosocial changes

        (3) Financial and legal implications

        (4) Interpersonal changes

        (5) Coping with behavioral outbursts

        (6) Need to change: transaction from feeling helpless to helping others

        (7) Debriefing and integration " . . . Have we done everything we could?"

        (8) Search for community alternatives

        (9) Crisis within the family

        (10) Sexuality

        (11) Anger toward outside group

        (12) Anger toward the patient

        (13) Love

        (14) Prospect of death

        (15) Bereavement

8. Management of patient and family with dementing illness

    a. Provision of information

    b. Direct care for medical and psychiatric problems

    c. Refer families to proper medical specialists

        d.   Refer families to community and health services
        e.   Assist family with institutionalization decision
        f.   Alert family to financial and legal advisors
        g.   Counsel family or refer for psychotherapy or family therapy
        h.   Obtain ongoing cognitive evaluation
        i.   Work with family to develop coping strategies
        j.   Refer families to self-help groups
        k.   Provide proper medication

C.   Depression
    1.   Facts and figures
        a.   Epidemiology
        b.   Causes of depressive disorders
        c.   Risk factors
    2.   Clinical manifestations of depression
        a.   Diagnostic challenge of older persons
        b.   Symptom dimensions
            (1) Affective
            (2) Behavioral
            (3) Somatic
            (4) Psychological
        c.   Medical diseases and drugs that can produce or exacerbate depression
    3.   Differential diagnosis
        a.   Clinical evaluation
        b.   Depressive categories
            (1) Existential sadness
            (2) Reactive depression
            (3) Unipolar depression
            (4) Bipolar depression
            (5) Schizoaffective disorders
    4.   Suicide
        a.   Risk factors
        b.   Management

    5. Treatment of depression
        a. Psychotherapy
        b. Pharmacotherapy
        c. ECT
        d. Combined approaches

D. Anxiety Disorders
    1. Anxiety in the aged
        a. Terminology
        b. Theories and methods
        c. Stress and anxiety
    2. Clinical manifestations of anxiety
        a. Impact of aging on manifestation of anxiety
            (1) Sympathetic nervous system changes
            (2) Physical illness
        b. Anxiety and CNS diseases
    3. Diagnosis of anxiety
        a. Subtypes of anxiety and effectiveness of treatment
        b. Disease vs. problems of living
        c. History: the best tool
        d. Psychometric ratings
        e. Psychophysiological assessment
    4. Management of treatment
        a. Development of a deliberate therapeutic plan
        b. Building support mechanisms for the patient
        c. Anxiety and depression
        d. Drug treatment
        e. Behavioral management
        f. Management in the long-term care facility

E. Paranoid Disorders
    1. Evaluation of paranoia
        a. Special issues, e.g., nutrition, sensory deficits
        b. Suspiciousness
        c. Transient paranoid reaction

        d.   Paraphrenia (late onset paranoia without schizophrenic illness)

        e.   Paranoia associated with schizophrenia of late onset

   2.   Treatment of suspiciousness and paranoia

        a.   Situational and environmental manipulation

        b.   Identification and replacement of loss

        c.   Observation

        d.   Psychopharmacologic strategies

        e.   Combined strategies

F.   Alcoholism and Drug Abuse

   1.   Issues in the study of alcohol abuse

        a.   Theories of alcoholism

           (1)   Psychological theories

              (a) Anxiety control

              (b) Learning theory

              (c) Personality disorders

              (d) Role modeling

              (e) Transactional theory

           (2)   Sociocultural theories

              (a) Culture specific

              (b) Subcultures under stress

              (c) Multiple losses

           (3)   Biological theories

              (a) Genetic

              (b) Biochemical

              (c) Endocrine

        b.   Measures of alcohol use and abuse

   2.   Issues in drug misuse and abuse among the aged

        a.   Data base in aging

        b.   Changing patterns as a function of changing economic status

        c.   Changing patterns as a function of health tolerance

   3.   Prescription misuse vs. illicit drug abuse

     a.   Older persons have more illness and receive more medications

     b.   Relationship between true need and pattern of drug use as a "way of life"

     c.   Compliance: Overuse and underuse

     d.   Ethical problems

     e.   Patient behavior

4.   Research on drug taking behavior

     a.   Individuality of drug use/misuse

     b.   Techniques for effective use and prevention of misuse of drugs

5.   Effective survey methods for study of substance abuse

     a.   Survey methods

     b.   Interview effects

     c.   Instrument effects

     d.   Respondent effects

6.   Management of alcoholism

     a.   Attitude toward older alcoholics

     b.   Resources deployed

     c.   Results of rehabilitation

     d.   Rehabilitation program

G.   Neurotic and Characterologic Disorders

1.   Personality adjustment/maladjustments during aging

     a.   Sociological orientation

        (1)   Developmental theories and life transitions

        (2)   Successful vs. unsuccessful aging

     b.   Psychiatric orientation

        (1)   Standards to measure adjustment

        (2)   Deviance

        (3)   Physical disability

2.   Overview of neurotic disorders in the aged

     a.   Lack of body of knowledge

        b. Prevalence
        c. Problems in definition of neurotic disorders
        d. Chronic neurotic disorder vs. late-life onset
        e. Higher mortality of neurotic older persons
        f. Psychometric evaluations of neuroticism
        g. Intellectual functioning of neurotic older persons

3. Loneliness and neurotic behavior
        a. Isolation vs. loneliness
        b. Types of loneliness
        c. Definition and management of loneliness
            (1) Psychiatric treatment for anxiety and depression
            (2) Medical intervention to improve health and capacity for socialization
            (3) Social intervention to improve socialization
4. Utilization of social services vs. medical intervention
5. Symptomatology of neurotic older person
        a. Hypochondriasis or high bodily concern
        b. Lifelong hypochondriasis
        c. Late-onset hypochondriasis as a predictor of suicide, depression, or physical illness
6. Etiology of neurotic disorder
        a. Vulnerable personality
        b. Life experience
        c. Stress and coping
        d. Impact of physical illness
7. Psychotherapy with neurotic disorders in later life

H. Sleep Disturbances
1. Age-related changes in sleep patterns
        a. Laboratory studies
            (1) REM (rapid eye movement)
            (2) Stage 4 sleep
            (3) Nocturnal awakenings

                (4)   Amount of sleep
          b.   Community surveys
      2.   Lack of data on nature of sleep disturbances in aged
          a.   Nomenclature of sleep disorders
          b.   Characteristics of sleep complaints in institutionalized aged
          c.   Characteristics of older insomniacs in community
          d.   Lifelong insomnia
          e.   Late-onset insomnia and brain changes
      3.   Utilization of sedatives/hypnotics
      4.   Management of sleep disturbances
          a.   Evaluation of sleep disturbances
                (1)   History of sleep disturbances
                (2)   Physical and psychiatric examinations
                (3)   Drug history
                (4)   Psychosocial history
                (5)   Sleep interview
                (6)   Referral to sleep disorder center
          b.   Assessment instrument
                (1)   Community residents
                (2)   Nursing home residents
           c.   Management of sleep disturbances
                (1)   Information about normal sleep changes with aging
                (2)   Impact of medical and psychiatric illness on sleep
                (3)   Behavioral management of sleep problems
                (4)   Recommendation for appropriate use of hypnotics
IV.   Management Strategies
    A.   Psychopharmacology: the Aging Patient/Client
      1.   Nomenclature of psychotropic drugs
          a.   Antipsychotic

       b.   Antidepressant
       c.   Antimanic
       d.   Antianxiety and hypnotics
       e.   Cognitive activity
2.   Side effects of medications on older persons
3.   Pharmacokinetics
       a.   Absorption
       b.   Distribution
       c.   Metabolism
       d.   Receptor state activity
       e.   Elimination
4.   Antipsychotic drugs
       a.   Therapeutic effects
       b.   Adverse effects
          (1)   Short-term
          (2)   Long-term
5.   Antidepressant drugs
       a.   Therapeutic effects
          (1)   Monoamine oxidase inhibitors
          (2)   Stimulants
          (3)   Tricyclic antidepressants
6.   Antimanic drugs
       a.   Efficacy of lithium
       b.   Toxicity of lithium complicated by management of concomitant illness
7.   Antianxiety drugs and hypnotics
       a.   Hypnotics
       b.   Benzodiazepines
8.   Cognitive-acting drugs
       a.   Rationale for drug therapy of cognitive dysfunction
       b.   Stimulants and analeptics
       c.   Vasodilators
       d.   Anticoagulants
       e.   Ergot alkaloids

       f.   RNA-like compounds
       g.   Gerovital
       h.   Hyperbaric oxygenation
       i.   Vitamins
       j.   Vasopressin
       k. β-Adrenergic blockers
       l.   Cholinergic drugs

B.   Behavioral Management
    1.   Overview
       a.   Need for more research about psychopathology
       b.   Data-based differential diagnosis necessary for therapeutic strategies
       c.   Individualized treatment
    2.   Development of treatment plan
       a.   Why treat?
       b.   Goals of treatment plan
       c.   Effect of environment on outcome
       d.   Special problems of cognitively impaired elderly
    3.   Therapeutic approaches
       a.   Contingency strategies
          (1) Speech and verbalization
          (2) Sensory-motor behavior
          (3) Self-care
          (4) Activity
          (5) Disruptive behavior
       b.   Reality orientation
       c.   Cognitive interventions
          (1) Cognitive enhancement/remediation
          (2) Locus of control
       d.   Psychosocial therapies
          (1) Supportive psychotherapy
          (2) Group therapy
          (3) Crisis intervention
       e.   Family therapy

        f.   Environmental interventions
            (1)   Perceived control
            (2)   Actual control

C.   Psychotherapy
   1.   Theoretical perspectives and their application
       a.   Psychoanalytic
       b.   Other psychodynamic schools
       c.   Counseling approaches
       d.   Nondirective
       e.   Directive
       f.   Cognitive
   2.   Historical development of geriatric psychotherapy
   3.   Strategies for psychotherapy
       a.   Brief therapy
       b.   Supportive therapy
       c.   Group therapies
       d.   Family therapies
       e.   Clinic intervention
   4.   Special issues in the approach to psychotherapy
       a.   Appropriate techniques
       b.   Transference
       c.   Authority of therapist
       d.   Combined drug-psychotherapy
       e.   Coordinating health team efforts
       f.   Dealing with chronic pain
       g.   Countertransference
       h.   Fear of death
       i.   Physical and interpersonal losses
   5.   Techniques for supportive therapy
       a.   Use of questions
       b.   Life review
       c.   Empathy
       d.   Removal of symptoms

      6. Self-help as an adjunct therapy
         a. Individuals
         b. Families
      7. Institutionally based therapies
D. Cognitive Training
      1. Rationale
         a. Cognitive enhancement for healthy older person
         b. Cognitive remediation for the cognitively impaired aged
      2. Measurement technology
         a. Microanalysis of behavior
         b. Assessment of change
      3. Foci for cognitive training
         a. Language
            (1) Expressive functions
            (2) Receptive functions
         b. Nonverbal communication
         c. General cognitive processes
            (1) Coding
            (2) Organizing
            (3) Rehearsing
            (4) Retrieving
         d. Attentional systems
            (1) Improvements in ability to focus attention
            (2) Improvements in ability to divide attention
         e. Memory system
            (1) Improvements in strategies and plans
            (2) Changes in executive function
            (3) Increases in knowledge base
      4. Principles of cognitive retraining
         a. Use existing abilities to strengthen impaired abilities

        b.   Use tasks with a hierarchy of difficulty
5.   Training family members and caregivers to do cognitive training
6.   Motivation and cognitive success
7.   Cognitive enhancement modules
        a.   Healthy older persons
        b.   Mildly impaired older persons
        c.   Moderately impaired older persons
        d.   Severely impaired older persons
8.   Designing a cognitively stimulating environment

E.   Sexual Counseling
1.   Factors relevant to understanding sexual activity in older persons
        a.   Demography
        b.   Belief system
           (1)   Desire to conform
           (2)   Values, norms, religious background
           (3)   Age of partner
        c.   Social and economic resources
           (1)   Availability of partner
           (2)   Social integration
        d.   Physical health
        e.   Emotional health
           (1)   Adaptation to aging
           (2)   Emotional disorders
        f.   Present sexual expression
           (1)   Sexually active
           (2)   Sexually expressive in other ways
           (3)   Sexual deviance
        g.   Prior patterns of sexual expression
        h.   Knowledge
           (1)   Changes in reproductive system
           (2)   Sexuality

2. Diagnostic evaluation
    a. Patient complaints
    b. Physical exam (including genitals)
    c. Drug history (current medications and dosage)
    d. Sexual history
        (1) Sexual activity
        (2) Masturbation
        (3) Erections
    e. Psychosocial history
        (1) Availability of partners
        (2) Marital conflicts
        (3) Communication patterns
        (4) Loneliness
        (5) Grief
        (6) Multiple losses
3. Outcome
    a. Sexual enhancement
    b. Sex therapy
4. Treatment objectives
    a. Provision of information
    b. Counseling
    c. Referral
F. Self-help Groups
    1. Overview of functions of local family support organizations
        a. Direct family support
            (1) Existence
            (2) Information, advice, and referral
            (3) Crisis intervention
            (4) Facilitation of small group formation
            (5) Home visits to individuals and couples
            (6) Long-term care counseling
            (7) Establishment of counseling services

      b. Interface with professional and community service
        (1) Medical/psychiatric counseling
        (2) Financial counseling
        (3) Community services
      c. Education
        (1) Professionals
        (2) Community

2. How groups are started and structured
    a. Help-seeking and self-help groups
      (1) Why the dementia self-help group movement started
      (2) Reasons for joining self-help groups
      (3) Self-help: Alternative to or preparation for psychotherapy?
    b. Self-help group development
      (1) Organization size
      (2) Organizational structure
      (3) Program focus
      (4) Nature of membership
      (5) Nature of leadership
      (6) Interfacing with professionals and agencies

3. Maintenance of self-help group
    a. Critical mass of patients and families
    b. Common setting: hospital, community
    c. Publicity
    d. Legitimacy
    e. Recruitment process
    f. Involvement of members

4. Mechanisms of change
    a. How self-help groups aid their members
      (1) Group cohesiveness (belonging to group)
      (2) Universality (learning that others have same problems)

          (3) Guidance (group members advising things to do and try)

          (4) Catharsis

          (5) Hope (seeing others solving similar problems)

          (6) Existential factors (recognizing that life is unjust at times)

          (7) Identification (finding someone in group to pattern after)

    b. How self-help groups could help their members more

          (1) Interpersonal learning

          (2) Coping with crisis

    c. Participant perceptions and what is helpful in self-help groups

          (1) Ideology

          (2) Professional leadership

          (3) Small face-to-face groups

          (4) Nature of the dementing illness

5. Setting up therapeutic family support group programs

    a. Group formation

    b. Family assessment

    c. Contracts

    d. Designing a program

    e. Role of consultants

    f. Role of family

G. The Institutional Environment

1. Issues in the decision to institutionalize

    a. Types of long-term care institutions

          (1) Nursing homes

          (2) State hospitals

          (3) Intermediate care facilities

          (4) Home

2. Long-term care facilities as a social system
    a. Societal need for long-term care institutions
    b. Goals, structure, and function
    c. Characteristics and roles of staff
    d. Characteristics and roles of residents
3. Institutional ecology
    a. Size
    b. Architecture and furnishings
    c. Psychosocial climate
4. The institution in the community
    a. Physical
    b. Social
    c. Legal
5. Impact of the relocation of residents
6. Potential for institutional change
7. Quality of care
8. Deinstitutionalization
9. Long-term care decisions
    a. Making a decision
        (1) Assessing patients' level of functioning
        (2) Assessing families' level of functioning
        (3) Evaluating socioeconomic resources
        (4) Evaluating community-based services
    b. Assessing the quality of a nursing home
        (1) Low staff turnover
        (2) Presence of volunteers
        (3) Individualized diets
        (4) Evidence of psychological therapies
        (5) Evidence of careful use of drugs and appropriate monitoring
        (6) Presence of rehabilitation programs and necessary equipment

       (7)   Presence of bowel and bladder training programs

       (8)   Evidence of exercise program for all residents

       (9)   Evidence of social activities

      (10)   Existence of resident councils and committees

      (11)   Indication of active, warm, concerned administrator and head nurse

      (12)   Availability of religious services

      (13)   Obvious evidence of personal freedom and choice

H.   Alternatives to Nursing Home Care

   1.   Health care assessment

      a.   Physical and mental health

      b.   Sensory acuity

      c.   Mobility and need for special aids

      d.   Economics

      e.   Personal and social support system

   2.   Health services delivery system

      a.   Identification of service

      b.   Delivery and coordination of services

      c.   Role of professionals

   3.   Alternatives to nursing homes

      a.   Day care

      b.   Home health

      c.   Organized home care

      d.   Intermediate housing

      e.   Day hospitals

      f.   Home help

   4.   Support for individual and family

I.   Community-based Comprehensive Care
  1. Overview
      a. Available services
      b. Limited access (lack of knowledge, finances, acceptability, mobility)
      c. Fragmented clinical and community services
  2. Objectives of community-based care
      a. Education of peer advocates
      b. Education of older persons to understand aging and chronic illness
      c. Creation/integration of services
      d. Case management
  3. Assessment of needs
      a. Demographic and socioeconomic
      b. Perceived health and need for services
      c. Present knowledge of services
      d. Present use of services
      e. Satisfaction with availability and accessibility of services
      f. Physical and mental health
  4. A program of comprehensive health care
      a. Intensive care
      b. Acute hospital care
      c. Subacute hospital care
      d. Ambulatory care
      e. Chronic care
      f. Centers where services can be delivered to healthy outpatients
      g. Group living accommodations for the healthy elderly
      h. Individual residences for the healthy elderly
  5. Services
      a. Medical screening and counseling

      b. Dental screening

      c. Drug counseling

      d. Nursing care, including podiatry

      e. Physician care

      f. Mental health counseling

6. Model programs

      a. Innovative outreach services

          (1) Shopping centers

          (2) Outreach professionals

          (3) Older outreach workers

      b. Information and assistance programs

          (1) Personal vs. telephone

          (2) Mobile vs. stationary

      c. Homebound services

      d   Innovative use of traditional health care services

          (1) Hospital-based home care program

          (2) Home health services provided by nursing homes

          (3) Health and mental health clinics at congregate meal site

      e. New approaches for health education and prevention

          (1) Multiphasic screening combined with health education

          (2) Radio health education

      f. Programs tailored to needs of minority aged

          (1) Specialized homemaker/home aide service

          (2) Language issues

7. Potential community services

      a. Home repair or chore services

      b. Homemaker or home health services

      c. Home delivered meals

      d. Group meals

  e. Senior centers or recreational care programs
  f. Telephone visiting and checking services
  g. Employment services
  h. Information and referral services
  i. Legal services
  j. Telephone bill assistance
  k. Laundry services
  l. Communication services for sight/hearing-impaired
  m. Visiting nurse service
  n. At-home physical therapy
  o. Counseling for emotional disturbances
 8. Why spend money and time on the frail elderly?

J. Care of the Dying Patient
 1. Patient attitudes
  a. Desire to be informed
  b. Loss of relationships
  c. Home vs. hospital
  d. Fear of dying
  e. Coping with death and coping with life
 2. Attitudes of health care professionals
  a. Avoid direct involvement
  b. Elderly less valuable than young
  c. Patient behavior determines care
  d. Training provides technical but not psychological skills
 3. Treatment of dying persons
  a. Goals
   (1) Maintain life as a human being
   (2) Maintain roles and identity
   (3) Monitor and treat depression
   (4) Monitor affect in patient and self
  b. Prevent indignity and isolation
  c. Discuss important decisions honestly

      d. Deal with patients' needs when and as they occur

      e. Behavior of professionals comfortable for dying patients
          (1) Draws from personal experience with terminal illness
          (2) Informs patient and family when diagnosis is certain
          (3) Provides information when patient requests
          (4) Assures patient that he/she will not be deserted
          (5) Continues contact with patient

  4. The process of dying
      a. The patient
      b. The family
      c. The doctor and health professional
      d. Who owns the patient?

  5. Principles of care
      a. Medical and psychosocial functions
      b. Care of dying is active treatment
      c. Hospice care
          (1) Admission
          (2) Personalized environment
          (3) Patient's symptoms are primary concern
          (4) Maintenance of alert, active human being
          (5) Psychiatric support for patients, family, staff
          (6) Prevent isolation
          (7) Philosophy: To live and die

V. Health Care Policy Issues
  A. Health Strategies for the Aged
    1. Overview of health care needs of aged
    2. Health maintenance

a. Government policy
b. Individual responsibility
3. Obstacles to health care
   a. Legal–political bureaucratic organization
   b. Financial
   c. Geographic
   d. Education and attitude of patient
   e. Education and attitude of health care professionals
   f. Absence of a system for continuity of care
4. Nursing homes and long-term care
   a. Nursing home: resource or warehouse?
   b. Alternatives to nursing homes
   c. Long-term care planning
5. Strategies for improving health care
   a. Training
   b. Demonstration model units
      (1) Family geriatric centers
      (2) Hospice
      (3) Cognitive enhancement center
      (4) Respite care
   c. Health care policy and strategy study centers
   d. Public information
6. Integration of health and other human services
B. Federal Policy Directions in Long-term Care
   1. Definition of long-term care
      a. Is related to functional limitations
      b. Recognizes wide range of individual needs
      c. Includes health, housing, personal and social service, and income maintenance
      d. Implies continuity of care, including prevention, acute care, as well as continuous care
      e. Requires many types of providers and both community and institution-based care

    2. Policy issues
- a. No consensus about public responsibility for long-term care
- b. Difficult to establish criteria for defining need for services
- c. Long-term care services are provided and financial aid limited by medical criteria
- d. Lack of social and community health care services to balance institutional care
- e. Wide variation in service availability and financing
- f. Coordination of multiple human service

    3. Objectives of long-term care
- a. Maximization of functional independence within limits of individual's impairment
- b. Rehabilitation
- c. Provision of care in the least restrictive environment possible
- d. Humane care for permanently dependent persons
- e. Death with dignity

    4. Alternatives for future of federal long-term care policy
- a. Improvement and coordination of existing resources
- b. Establishment of a separate federal long-term care benefit program
- c. Provision of additional income to consumers
- d. Initiation of long-term care developments in the private sector

C. Recent Long-term Care Policy Recommendations and Legislative Proposals
    1. Recommendations in *Home Health and Other In-House Service: Titles XVIII, XIX, XX of the Social*

Security Act, A Report to Congress, HEW, October 1979.

2. *Recommendations in Public Policy of the Frail Elderly,* A Staff Report to the Federal Council on Aging, HEW, December 1978.

3. *The Medicaid Community Care Act of 1980,* (H.R. 6194).

4. *The Medicare Long Term Care Act of 1979,* (H.R. 58).

5. *Title XXI—Comprehensive Community Bond Non-Institutional Long Term Care Service for the Frail and Disabled.*

6. Medicare Amendments of 1980 (H.R. 3990)

7. Medicare and Medicaid Amendments of 1981 (Titles A, B, and C of Title XXI).

D.   Long-term Care in Other Countries

1.   England

    a.   Reorganization of national health service in 1974

    b.   Regional provision of services

    c.   Competition of aged with other interest groups for funds

    d.   Provision of free medical care

       (1)   Physicians paid by number of patients

       (2)   Higher fee paid for older patients

    e.   Institutionalization as a last resort

       (1)   Home philosophically desirable

       (2)   Shortage of residential and hospital beds

       (3)   Home services cost effective

    f.   Home care delivered by health visitors, home nurses, midwives

    g.   Trend toward health center practice by physicians

    h.   Most hospitals have geriatric assessment units

    i.   Innovative approach

      (1)   Group housing with case manager or "warden"

      (2)   Five day ward, weekend home

   j.   Philosophy of "making do" with limited resources

   k.   Volunteer services important

2.   Scotland

   a.   Geriatric care more popular than pediatrics

   b.   Deliberate planning

      (1)   Goal of 25 residential beds per 1,000 aged

      (2)   Residential care with personalized care

   c.   Ideal care

      (1)   Home maintenance

      (2)   Health center as nucleus of care

      (3)   Health visitors

      (4)   Warden housing

      (5)   Respite care

   d.   Health system in transition

      (1)   Volunteers

      (2)   Attitudes

3.   Sweden

   a.   National pension plan

   b.   Health care and social welfare are local responsibilities

   c.   Hospital and institutional care predominate

      (1)   Beds increasing

      (2)   Home care limited to low-paid home-helpers

      (3)   Shortage of nursing home beds

      (4)   National Board of Health imposes few regulations on nursing homes

   d.   Long-term care system

      (1)   10% of people in hospitals or clinics for diagnosis

          (2)   30% in central nursing homes for active rehabilitation

          (3)   60% in local nursing homes for chronic illnesses

4. Norway
   a. Philosophy: to enhance individual autonomy
   b. Individual absorbs health care cost
   c. Primary care centers developing regionally
   d. Municipalities provide home helpers, meals, transportation
   e. Institutional care growing

5. Netherlands
   a. Care of aged under four ministries
      (1) Public health (hospitals and nursing homes)
      (2) Housing (old age homes and residential dwellings)
      (3) Culture, recreational, and social work (service centers)
      (4) Social affairs (sick funds, insurance plans)
      (5) Interministerial council coordinated services
   b. Institutional care growing
   c. Special housing for aged

6. Israel
   a. Kupat Holim provides more acute care than long-term care
   b. Shortage of high-quality long-term care beds
      (1) Government has established five-star rating system for quality center
      (2) Cultural homogeneity emphasized
   c. Mishnan and the healthy aged
   d. Malben established to provide services for immigrants

e. Service for the Aging established 1967 by Minis-
    try of Health
    (1) Strengthens communities of aged
    (2) Aged encouraged to participate
f. Housing inadequate for aged
g. Home services inadequate for aged

5
A Framework for Curriculum Evaluation

Evaluation of an education program requires a conceptual model, goals, and a set of objective standards. Although specific objectives can be identified for each mental health specialty and in turn for individual programs, some objectives should be met by all program components. Theoretically, an increased knowledge base, supervised experience in clinical skills, and more positive attitudes toward rehabilitation of the aged should result in the development of more accomplished clinicians and better-quality care for the older patient. The specific knowledge, skills, and attitudes to be developed are reviewed in chapter 2.

A model for evaluation adapted from Perry (1980) and Shortell and Richardson (1978) provides a useful framework for the evaluation of a curriculum for training mental health professionals to care for the aged. Elements of the model are presented in Table 5.1. These include: (1) antecedent conditions, i.e., the existence of target patient and professional populations; (2) a set of program components, i.e., objectives, resources, and activities; (3) a set of intervening variables, e.g., changing funds, faculty, and curriculum; and (4) a set of outcome variables to evaluate the impact of the program, e.g., better health care system for the aging and aged, greater patient satisfaction, greater health provider satisfaction, increased use of professional agencies, and improved organizational collaboration.

This model includes an evaluation of both the implementation of training components and the impact of the curriculum. The

TABLE 5.1

A Process Model for Training Evaluation of Mental Health Professionals.
Adapted from Perry (1980), and Shortell and Richardson (1978).

ANTECEDENT CONDITIONS	PROGRAM COMPONENTS	INTERVENING VARIABLES	IMPACT
1. Target population of older patients.	1. Program objectives a) Improved interviewing, diagnostic, and treatment skills. b) Improved knowledge of aging and clinical aspects of aging. c) Improved attitudes towards rehabilitation of aged. d) Basic research and evaluation skills. e) Improved curriculum and program.	1. Program funding. 2. Changes in faculty. 3. Changes in clinical training sites. 4. Changes in curriculum.	1. Better health care system for the aged. 2. Greater patient satisfaction. 3. Greater health care provider satisfaction. 4. Improved collaboration among professionals, organizations. 5. Improved delivery and quality of hospital-based care. 6. Improved delivery and quality of community-based care. 7. Improved strategies for diagnosis and treatment.
2. Mental health professionals.	2. Program resources a) Professional and medical schools. b) Divisions of aging. c) Institute on aging. d) Faculty role models. e) Clinical sites. f) Community agencies. g) Admissions and supervisory committee.		
	3. Program activities a) Educational opportunities: didactics, seminars, patient care conferences. b) Clinical supervision. c) Individual and program evaluation. d) Opportunities for advanced training, research, policy discussions.		

general goals are to evaluate the extent to which the program is implemented as well as the success of the program as perceived by faculty and students; to develop and apply measures of the quality of student performance; and to evaluate student performance over time as an approximate measure of the effectiveness of the program.

Program and curriculum evaluations can be very simple or quite complicated. It is important that any decisions about the evaluation design be made early in the development of a training program. It is also necessary that the evaluation procedure be tailored to the individual institution, program, or discipline involved. We propose here a three-phase evaluation design to evaluate accomplishments of students as well as the success of the overall curriculum. Phase I examines how well the program is implemented as well as the perceptions of faculty and students. Phase II examines cognitive and attitudinal changes at the completion of curriculum units or days, weeks, months, or years of training. Phase III measures performance through chart audits and reviews. Our discussion of curriculum evaluation is not a sophisticated analysis, but there are a variety of conceptual and empirical studies in the literature for the interested reader (Bernstein, Bohrnstedt, & Borgatta, 1975; Cain, 1975; Campbell & Stanley, 1966; Riedel & Riedel, 1979; Shortell & Richardson, 1978; Weiss, 1972).

PHASE I

Detailed evaluations are collected from faculty, staff, students, and patients to determine the success of clinical experiences, lectures, seminars, and research activities. Sample evaluation forms for clinical, educational, and research activities throughout the training program for mental health professionals are found in Appendix I.

Evaluation in Phase I requires the formation of a faculty decision-making committee to monitor performance, as well as to develop and/or enforce standards for training credentials awarded at the completion of training. Of course, several decision-making groups on various levels should exist in addition to faculty committees: students, faculty, staff at clinical and community training sites, professional schools sponsoring the training, and funding agencies. Evaluation of training by each of these groups is important for the success of a training program, and each group requires specific information to evaluate the quality of the training experience (Table 5.2).

PHASE II

Phase II procedures involve the comparison of pretraining and posttraining test performance. The aim of Phase II is to identify changes in knowledge about aging, diagnostic and treatment modalities, health care systems, and policy implications, as well as changes in attitudes. Evaluation tools may include written as well as oral examinations, given both informally and formally. Several tests have been designed to evaluate changes in attitudes toward older persons and their clinical care (Hickey, Rakowski, & Hultsch, 1976; Holtzman, Beck, Hodgetts, Coggan, & Ryan, 1978; Kilty & Feld, 1976; Kogan, 1961; Rosencrantz & McNevin, 1969; Tuckman & Lorge, 1953; Weinberger & Milham, 1975).

PHASE III

Phase III procedures attempt to identify performance changes in the trainee. They focus on interactions with and treatment of older patients. Tools for judging performance are direct observation, supervisor's reports, and chart reviews. (See Appendix for sample evaluation forms.) Specifically evaluated are the individual's diagnostic acumen, adequacy of functional and psychosocial assessments, psychopharmacologic knowledge, ability to identify and use community resources, ability to make referrals, and effectiveness in choosing appropriate management and treatment strategies. It may be worthwhile to discuss the choice of instruments with the students, particularly those at an advanced level.

TABLE 5.2

Decision-making Groups Important for Evaluation of the Success and Effectiveness of Training for Mental Health Professionals in Aging. Adapted from Perry (1980).

DECISION-MAKING GROUPS

TIME COURSE		STUDENTS	FACULTY	FACULTY AND STAFF AT TRAINING SITES	PROFESSIONAL SCHOOL	FUNDING AGENCY
BEFORE TRAINING	DECISION	Enroll or not.	Training objectives and content. Methods of evaluations.	Time and effort required. Number of patients needed.		
	DATA SOURCES	Training requirements, prior evaluations.	Literature and other programs.	Faculty.		
DURING TRAINING	DECISION	Where and how to focus training to maximize learning.	How to ensure quality learning experiences and opportunities.	How to be of most help to students.		
	DATA SOURCES	Evaluations by faculty, staff, and patients.	Evaluations by students, other faculty, staff, and patients.	Evaluation and feedback from students, other faculty, staff, and patients.		
AFTER TRAINING	DECISION	Get more training? See more older patients in practice?	How to record student competence, evaluate training impact. Any curriculum changes?	Changes to make?	How much curriculum time?	Continue funds? New programs to fund?
	DATA SOURCES	Own experience from training, feedback, and encouragement from faculty.	Written and oral exams, attitude measures, evaluations from students, faculty, and staff.	Evaluations from students, faculty, staff, and patients.	Training evaluations by faculty, students, staff, and patients.	All evaluation measures.

II
Concepts and Issues
in Training

6
Overview of Mental Health Care for Older Persons: A Critique

During the 1950s and early 1960s approximately one-quarter of all first admissions to state hospitals were for patients aged 65 and older, and half of all state hospital populations were in this age group. Only two percent of the psychiatric outpatient care was delivered to the aged during this period. Indeed, the delivery of mental health care could be best described as "all-or-none"; older persons received little preventive or outpatient therapeutic care and were at a heightened risk for long-term custodial placement.

This all-or-none response pattern changed somewhat during the late sixties because of the transfer of the aged from state hospitals to nursing homes and other long-term care facilities. The shift was a consequence of the reduced cost of care in facilities other than state hospitals due to the availability of partial reimbursement in such alternative settings. As the nature of the facility changed, old problems became even more acute. Direct admissions from the community rarely involved mental health evaluations, and the shift took place with no provisions to determine level of psychiatric services needed for nursing home inpatient care or mental health intervention. The result was the development of nursing home warehouses with a poor level of care.

Between 1963 and 1967, the resident population of nursing homes increased to 756,000, with 186,000 identified as mentally ill patients. By 1967 there were more mentally ill aged in nursing homes than in psychiatric inpatient facilities. The trend has continued, and now many nursing homes are mini-mental hospitals, while many state hospitals are denying admission to older psychiatric patients. The problem is complicated by the failure of most nursing homes to have any identifiable, ongoing psychiatric care. Greater reliance has been placed on "tranquilizing" and sedating psychotropic medication in an attempt to ease the burden of patient management for the staff. Thus, the vast majority of nursing home patients in the United States are on such drugs.

Approximately 4.5 percent of persons over age 65 are now in institutions. Conservative estimates indicate that a minimum of 60 percent of these residents have psychiatric disorders, yet the diagnostic assessment of them is woefully inadequate. And despite a high proportion of older psychiatrically impaired patients in nursing homes (90% of patients in nursing homes are over age 65), outpatient psychiatric clinics still devote only 2 percent of their services to the elderly. Federally subsidized community mental health centers have a slightly better record, with 4 percent of their services being delivered to the aged.

Although persons 65 years and older comprise a significant proportion of the population and are at high risk for mental illness, the data continue to indicate an all-or-none approach to the solution of their mental health problems. Most of our professional resources are diverted to a custodial system instead of a community-based system for diagnosis, treatment, or referral. Lacking adequate health services to detect the early manifestations of mental or emotional disorders, we are creating a cadre of more seriously affected older persons who will require still more intensive care. The problem, however, does not lie solely in the attitude of professionals toward older patients. Older persons and their families frequently deny mental health problems and avoid intervention or care which may be characterized as "psychiatric."

As the proportion of the aged continues to increase, many significant problems will worsen. The heightened prevalence of cognitive and emotional disturbances, with the associated need for care for frail older patients, is a major issue. The emphasis on custodial instead of outpatient care for impaired older persons constitutes another significant focus for concern, as does the absence of a therapeutic orientation, in or out of institutions. Finally, the difficulty of finding qualified personnel to understand and serve the needs of the aged is clearly fundamental.

The application of research findings to patient care has received much rhetoric but little support in recent years. There is, for example, a "hopeless" attitude assigned to brain disorders in later life, as well as a misconception that all older persons will show progressive loss. These are unsubstantiated by data from longitudinal studies for persons through age 75. The belief that such decline will lead to nonreversible dementing illness and psychosis is also not supported by the available data.

Loss of the capacity to think, learn, or remember is one of the most dreaded aspects of growing old. Unfortunately, the term *senility* has come to be commonly used to describe these losses. "Senility" should be discarded from the professional lexicon because its use advances at least two misconceptions: that inevitable mental changes occur with advancing age, and that nothing can be done for persons suffering such changes. This is simply not true. It is a mistake to assume that normal aging is characterized by a profound and progressive decline in intellectual functions and abilities (Cohen & Wu, 1980; Eisdorfer, 1978; Jarvik, Eisdorfer, & Blum, 1973; Labouvie-Vief, 1980; Schaie, 1977–8).

Changes in personality and intellect occur in many older people, but aging per se may not be the basis for the pathology seen. If an older person shows signs of cognitive or emotional disturbances, it is important to evaluate whether there are treatable causes of the decline (Eisdorfer & Cohen, 1978; Libow, 1973; Wells, 1979). Infections, metabolic disorders, poor nutritional habits, circulatory and pulmonary diseases, drug effects, social isolation, depression, and alcohol and drug abuse are all possible causes of intellectual change. A number of factors other than health have a significant impact on behavior. These include motivation, feelings of self-worth and competence, the ability to work or use time effectively, finances, independence, mobility, and experience.

Not all intellectual changes are reversible. There is a group of brain diseases in which intellectual functioning, personality, and the ability for self-care deteriorate progressively in middle-aged and older adults (Eisdorfer & Cohen, 1978, 1980; Katzman & Karasu, 1975). These include metabolic and vascular disorders, hypoxia and anoxia (lack of oxygen), nutritional deficiency, alcohol and drug abuse, toxic substances such as metals (lead, mercury) and carbon monoxide, brain tumors, trauma (head injuries, heat strokes), infections, and a variety of such diseases as multiple sclerosis (Wells, 1977). Other diseases of the central nervous system whose primary symptoms are dementia include Alzheimer's disease, Pick's disease, Huntington's chorea, Parkinson's disease, and Creutzfeld-Jacob's disease.

Alzheimer's disease is the most common form of dementing illness, affecting more than 50 percent of all people with dementia (Tomlinson, Blessed, & Roth, 1970). The second most important disorder, accounting for another 20 percent, is vascular dementia, also known as multi-infarct dementia; it is due to multiple small strokes. The remaining 30 percent are affected by "mixed" dementias, Pick's disease, alcoholism, multiple sclerosis, Huntington's chorea, viruses, metabolic diseases, and head trauma.

Although dementing illness affects 10 to 20 percent of the aged over age 65, it is not the major problem of the aged. For most elderly in the community, depression is probably a more serious risk. Transient depression, often secondary to the loss of some valued person, object, or role, is not infrequent in older persons (Blazer & Williams, 1980; Gurland, 1976; Gurland, Dean, Cross, & Golden, 1980). Also constituting major problems are the recurrence of endogenous depression and the prevalence of episodes of depression secondary to illness or medications; such affective disturbances in older persons may manifest as insomnia, apathy, persistent pain, bowel disturbance, and other somatic disorders. Often only the medical or motivational symptoms of the depression are treated and the factors in the patient's life causing the depression are ignored. The physician may knowingly treat only the physical symptoms, feeling that the isolation and losses of the aged are a social problem, not a medical one.

Part of the problem of delivering mental health services to older persons is the lack of outpatient and preventive care programs, but also seriously lacking are therapeutic strategies in all settings, including long-term care facilities. There exists, insofar as the care of the aged is concerned, a spirit of therapeutic nihilism totally unwarranted by the data. In institutions where aggressive treatment approaches are taken with regressed patients, the results have almost always been successful. Indeed, almost any kind of treatment given today's elderly will result in some positive outcome.

The major barrier to care appears to be the discomfort of a large segment of mental health professionals in working with the aged. This discomfort has been ignored and has yielded an apparent lack of concern with treatment of the elderly, which in turn has led to a failure to employ therapeutic techniques and an attitude of unwarranted pessimism. The approach to the elderly paranoid patient is a case in point (Eisdorfer, 1980). Late-onset paranoid symptoms are treatable, and a consideration of the role of hearing loss, social isolation, and learned helplessness may contribute to our understanding and development of community-based care for the elderly with paranoid ideation.

As the life expectancy for older persons increases, the problems associated with clinical care of the aging mentally ill worsen. According to all epidemiologic studies, the need for care increases with age (Kramer, 1980). Indeed, the risk for nonreversible dementing illnesses appears to double every five years after age 60 (Kay, 1977). Life expectancy at age 65 is nearly 15 years, and a vigorous attack to decrease cardiovascular illness alone, if successful, would add an additional 10.4 years to life expectancy at age 65 (Brotman, 1980). The prospect of a mean life expectancy of approximately 90 years for persons reaching age 65 thus would substantially increase the need for psychiatric services of the elderly.

Kramer and co-workers estimated that the number of older persons needing professional mental health services in the United States in 1980 would range from 2.3 million to as many as 4.7 million individuals (Kramer, Taube, & Redick, 1973). Projecting from current data, however, only 352,000 would have had services available. Thus, only 15 percent of those aged requiring psychiatric or other professional mental health services would have been able to receive them in 1980. This gap will be at least as severe in 1990.

To conclude, the care of mentally ill older persons seems likely to become even more inadequate unless there are changes in policy. Care is now oriented toward institutional management rather than toward the individual and his/her needs for outpatient and community programs. The focus is on disease and crisis, rather than on prevention, maintenance, or remediation. The expectation of a deterioration of the patient prevents a proper emphasis on the interaction between the physical, social, and psychological needs of the patient.

This faulty approach is largely based upon a failure to study the problem or to develop new therapeutic or management programs. Given this pessimistic orientation, diagnosis may be seen as irrelevant and is often inadequately performed. The complicated symptoms presented by the aged, which may cross from the behavioral and social to the physical, the lack of continuity in the care system, and the lack of communication between mental health and physical health practitioners, all combine to make the care of the aged an especially difficult challenge. The challenge of quality care for the aged transcends professional boundaries.

7
Health versus Healing:
Health Care of
Older Persons

Demographic studies to date confirm the concept proposed by Gompertz in 1825: The older the individual, the more likely he or she is to die. Furthermore, the risk for major health problems increases with advancing age: age past adolescence is a direct correlate of the probability of chronic or acute disease and the need for medical care. The National Center for Health Statistics (Kovar, 1977) estimates that 81 percent of all persons in the United States over age 65 have some form of chronic illness. Possibly more significant, 45 percent of those over age 65 experience limitations due to these conditions, and 39.4 percent are limited in major activities. Of persons in the age group 45 to 64, 24.3 percent are estimated to have some limitation in activity, and 19.1 percent have major limitations. Furthermore, 20 percent of people over age 65 are not fully mobile: of these, 10 percent are bedridden; 25 percent are household bound; 35 percent move with assistance; and 30 percent move with difficulty (Kovar, 1977).

Expenditures for health care are becoming a significant burden, not only for older patients, but for society as well. Hospital costs have increased fivefold since 1950, and physician fees more than doubled between 1965 and 1975. A large proportion of the national economy, nearly 10 percent of the annual gross national product (more than $142.5. billion in fiscal year 1977) is being spent for health care (Kovar, 1977).

Whereas the aged comprise 11 percent of the population, they account for 30 percent of the total U.S. expenditures for personal health care costs (Gibson & Fisher, 1978). Per capita, persons aged 65 and over receive care in outpatient settings about 40 percent more often than younger adults, are admitted to hospitals about 2.5 times more often, spend 3 times as many hospital days, and account for well over 90 percent of the long-term care patients in the United States. In fiscal 1977, total expenditure for personal health care of older persons was $41.3 billion. Of this figure 67 percent ($27 billion) was paid by the public, and adjusting for Medicare payments, the public portion was 60 percent. Out-of-pocket expenses for older persons accounted for 35 percent of the figure, and personal health insurance absorbed 5 percent of the cost (Gibson & Fisher, 1978). Clearly, the cost of care for the older person is becoming a significant personal and national burden.

The rising number and proportion of older persons presents a significant challenge: to improve our knowledge about aging and the illness pattern of the aged, and to develop diagnostic and treatment strategies as well as programs for health promotion. The Institute of Medicine's Report on Aging and Medical Education (1978) emphasizes the strength of the current data base on aging and clinical aspects of aging. The illness pattern of the aged is different from that of the young. Older patients have multiple chronic problems, and the ability to cope effectively with these problems varies considerably among individuals (IOM, 1978). Chronic conditions are three to four times more frequent among individuals in nursing homes. Unfortunately, while a large proportion of the aged are in long-term care, the major locus of health care is the hospital, and the focus is on acute care or episodes of crisis.

CONCEPTUALIZATION OF HEALTH CARE
OF OLDER PERSONS

One of the central issues in health care in the United States is whether health care programs should be directed toward health or toward healing. Health care programs based on one or the other of these related goals result in very different government and private policies. Health is defined by Blakeston's *New Gould Medical Dictionary* as "the state of dynamic equilibrium between the organism and its environment which maintains the structural and functional characteristics of the organism within the normal limit for the particular form of life (race, genes, species), and the particular phase of its life cycle." The definition for healing is "the process or act of getting well or of making well; the restoration to normal. . . ." Thus, if health is the goal, activities and expenditures are invested to preserve an acceptable equilibrium between a person and his/her environment. If, on the other hand, healing is emphasized, programs aim to restore sick individuals (i.e., those who are defined by self or others as showing the signs or symptoms of pathology) to some more optimal state. Programs focused on health use strategies of public health, preventive medicine, and health maintenance, while those directed toward healing emphasize medical care and the health services delivery system.

Another key issue is the extent to which health is an individual matter versus the extent to which it is a public concern. Health maintenance is to a certain degree an individual matter involving personal patterns of diet, exercise, smoking, rest, and activity. Diseases of affluence and excess may pose as significant a set of problems to our society as do the diseases of poverty. Such phenomena as obesity (which leads to hypertension and cardiovascular illness), alcoholism, drug abuse, drug addiction, and accidents account for a very significant portion of adult disease and death. However, the community also has a major impact on health. Poverty and deprivation are major causes of illness. Race and economic status are important factors in calculating both infant mortality and life expectancy. Social and political activities are required to develop public health information programs as well as specific health services.

The balance between health as an individual concern in contrast to a public concern has been shifting. Questions about which stance should predominate are raised by the debate about fluoridation of water, the sanctity of the doctor–patient relationship, disclosure of privileged information, and the "right to health care." Until quite recently, the movement in the United States over the past several decades has been the assumption of a stronger voice by the federal government in the control of health hazards, e.g., smoking, drug abuse, and air and water pollution. Sometimes, the value of this control is clear: pure water or effective waste disposal, for example, are helpful to all members of the community. Sometimes, however, the need for governmental involvement may not be apparent, or at least may raise a series of complex legal, financial, and political issues. Examples are the control of alcohol, tobacco, drugs, and industrial wastes.

When a state or federal government or even the private sector assumes responsibility for the health care costs of a defined population—such as the aged—it is in the interests of that government (and the people who support it) to reduce the cost of care without impairing quality. One simple method of reducing costs is reducing the amount of health care necessary. Prevention of illness is less costly than diagnosis and treatment. Unfortunately, the efficacy of prevention is often obscure, and it is certainly less clear to the consumer (taxpayer) than its cost in dollars or in limitations on behavior (e.g., diet, exercise, limitation on pesticides, pollution controls). As a result, prevention programs have clear disincentives, while their rewards are not readily apparent.

Just as health is affected by a range of biopsychosocial factors, so do government health care programs overlap with social welfare programs. There are many programs defined as "health" related which can also be considered "social welfare" related. This has often led to administrative problems in the past. Unfortunately, the array of economic, housing, or social services necessary to maintain a person at home in lieu of institutionalization is not as readily accepted as a legitimate "health" care cost. The result may be that in an effort to reduce costs, programs which appear only marginally "health" related are eliminated from the health services provided by governments. This is a particularly important problem in the functional health care of older persons.

The cost of health care to the nation has emerged as the important underlying issue. Expenditures for all types of health and medical services have increased steadily for well over a decade.

Between fiscal 1960 and fiscal 1979, the expenditure for services alone rose from $24.2 billion to $200 billion. With the addition of research and construction costs, the fiscal year 1979 budget for all types of health care was many more billions of dollars. Perhaps more significantly, health care expenditures as a proportion of our gross national product increased from 5.2 to 9.5 percent between 1960 and 1979.

The largest proportional increment during this period was in nursing home care: from a $500 million expenditure in 1960 to a 1977 expenditure of $10.5 billion. Gibson and Fisher (1978) estimate that the total long-term care bill was closer to $30 billion since approximately $20 billion were spent in the acute care of chronic patients within the hospital (including physician costs). The Health Care Financing Administration (HCFA, 1981) recently projected a $75 billion budget for nursing home facilities in 1985.

In sharp contrast, Brody (1981) observed that the combined programs of the Administration on Aging, Department of Agriculture, Community Service Administration, Social Service Administration, and the Department of Administrative Services spent a total of one billion dollars for community health/social services for prevention and rehabilitation of the impaired aged. Thus, the ratio of medical expenditures to health/service expenditures for long-term support in the community was 30 to 1.

HEALTH MAINTENANCE

The prominent phenomenologic aspects of human frailty with advancing age have focused health care on diseases and disabilities. As a result, we have ignored the potential of programs emphasizing maintenance of ability and promotion of health. This neglect of health-promotion programs is partly due to general community attitudes, and it is partly a reflection of the attitude of physicians and other health professionals toward the aged. Physicians are oriented toward healing, and their relations with the aged who show pathology (in contrast, for example, with infants, who may not) reinforces this orientation. Also, burdened with the threat of liability and malpractice, the tendency is for the physician in private practice to treat and protect patients rather than to discharge them and develop individualized long-term health maintenance programs. A program of activity and independence rather than dependence and "pushing" individuals into activities is often seen as undesirable and dangerous by the physician. The attitude that the older person is no longer useful in society in conjunction with the frequently observed pattern of loneliness, isolation, and depression generate an additional set of problems in caring for older persons. Thus, physician reflecting society's attitudes, often show little desire to invest heavily in aged individuals, who are not "attractive" patients.

Government-sponsored programs do little to help older people with health maintenance through exercise, periodic health checks, or education about such issues as nutrition and dental care. Indeed, most older individuals have little understanding of appropriate expectations for their own health. Since the expectation shared by health professionals, the community, and older persons alike is that older individuals are likely to be sick, few resources have been invested in ways to keep them from becoming sick.

Expectation is an important, although complex, issue in health care. Using a semantic differential instrument designed to explore the implications of certain terms in common usage, data already exist to indicate that the concept of "old" is strongly associated with "sick". In contrast, if "old" is paired with such terms as "strong" and "health," the association becomes discordant and is less acceptable, not only to most young people, but also to a large number of older persons themselves. This expectation of illness in the aged has dramatic consequences for health services delivery.

One of the changes needed in United States health care policy is in our expectation of sickness in older persons. It must be recognized that although the current generation of older persons manifests illness at a high rate, there is no justification for a long-term strategy ignoring the potential value of programs to prolong activity and maintain good health. Indeed, for the most affluent in our culture, attempts to "prevent" aging already exist. There is a large market in cosmetics purporting to restore youthful appearance and rejuvenating products of one sort or another.

In the absence of changing attitudes as well as greater investments in the health maintenance of older persons, we could create unnecessary health hazards for incoming waves of older individuals. Current attitudes may be contributing to the prevalence of sickness among the aged. For example, when older persons suffer from heart attacks, far less is usually done to return them to optimal function than is done for the general population. Little effort is invested to explore activities, needs, and interests with the older person. For many decades, physicians have been advising older persons with post-myocardial infarction to "eliminate" sexual activities on the assumption that sex was of little consequence to older adults. Only in the last decade have attitudes in some sectors changed with increasing information about the sexual interests and activities of older persons. The near alcoholism of many older Americans is ignored as it is assumed that they have little to do other than drink. Physical care of the older individual emphasizes pathology and minimal recovery, with little investment in prevention or full restoration. The need for the development of a strong program of positive health improvement and maintenance for older persons is clear.

8
Continuity of Care and the Present Nature of Long-term Care

A comprehensive program providing continuity of care for older persons in the United States is lacking. A patchwork of individual services exists, and each service is under a different management. Indeed, health care in the United States has been described as a cottage industry characterized by individual entrepreneurs. There are thousands of agencies providing homemaker and home health aid in the United States, and typically they comprise a series of discrete, competitive facilities in the same community, rather than a network of integrated health care services.

Services have been tied to a variety of financing mechanisms, such as Medicare, Medicaid, SSI, Title XX, and OAA, and this has compounded the patchwork nature of services. Policies differ about who should be served and the conditions for being served. Some units provide services to individuals with support from a city, county, or state. Many are private, both for profit and nonprofit. Some utilize federal monies directly, while others are covered by third-party carriers or state packages. The result of this patchwork financing is that "the flow of care of the aged follows the dollar," as Margaret Blenkner (1967) has accurately stated. For example, people are kept in institutions since services provided in an institution are reimbursed under Medicare or Medicaid while similar services provided in the home are not reimbursed. Historically, the decrease in the number of residents in mental hospitals was related to the increased use of nursing homes and other facilities when Medicaid dollars paid for care in the latter but not the former.

Another example of our failures in providing care for the aged involves rehabilitation programs. The elderly receive little help from such state and federal programs. Only 1 percent of rehabilitation dollars are spent for older persons.

Health maintenance organizations (HMOs) serve millions of Americans, but only a minority of all Americans live within HMO regions. In the past, the federal administration proposed a large increase in HMOs in order to enroll the vast majority of older Americans. Different HMOs, however, have different policies toward the aged, and many would provide no specialized services to older patients. Examples of specialized services valuable to the aged include community-based care, information and counseling services, geriatric outpatient clinics, day-care programs, halfway houses, rehabilitation centers and senior citizen centers.

NURSING HOMES AND LONG-TERM CARE

Initially, either county "poor farms," religious "old-age homes," or small private boarding homes served to care for the aged. Many of these facilities were operated on a profit-making basis by untrained individuals, and most were custodial rather than health oriented; many would not accept sick persons. Thus, the nursing home industry was rooted in the boarding home rather than the hospital tradition. It was not until 1940 to 1950 that licensing programs for nursing homes were adopted, and even in the early Fifties, most lacked skilled nursing and medical personnel as well as therapeutic services. The Kerr-Mills bill in 1961 legislated the allocation of federal matching funds to those states which established licensing and inspection programs for nursing homes. Until then, the nursing home was not considered a significant part of the health services system. Members of the health profession generally ignored these (profit-oriented) custodial facilities. Nursing homes were considered lodgings for those who could not care for themselves or receive care at home, i.e., the isolated and frail aged rather than patients requiring therapy.

In the Fifties, a number of factors led to a change in the status of the nursing home. Older persons increased in number and proportion in the population. Increasing urbanization led to a reduction in personal home facilities available for older persons and decreased the number of families able to care for their aged relatives within a single family dwelling. Incentives under the Kerr-Mills Act and the higher average income of older persons began to play a role. But perhaps the most significant change occurred in the mid-Sixties with the Medicare/Medicaid Legislation in 1965 and 1967; it not only provided for an improvement in nursing home standards but also substantially increased apparent incentives to nursing home care.

A number of different facilities may be called nursing homes. These include the Extended Care Facility (ECF), primarily designed to support post-hospital therapy with short-term, high-quality rehabilitative care; the skilled nursing facility (SNF), designed to provide less intensive long-term care than the ECF; and the Intermediate Care Facility (ICF), which provides maintenance and limited supportive nursing care, but not "skilled nursing" services.

Although there are slight differences in statistics depending upon the types of nursing homes included in the analysis, it is clear that there was an increase of more than 100 percent in the number of long-term care beds available between 1963 and 1970. If nursing home and related care facilities such as Intermediate Care Facilities are included, then between 1963 and 1974, the increase was from 319,000 to about 1,100,000 beds. SSA Amendments of 1967 provided for the establishment under Title XI of Intermediate Care Facilities, which caused a growth of such units exceeding that of nursing homes. Long-term care beds have continued to increase, and the National Nursing Home survey (National Center for Health Statistics, 1979) showed that there were 1,303,000 residents in 18,900 homes in 1977, a 21 percent increase since 1974. Skilled nursing facilities are the most common facility, followed by intermediate care and a combination of skilled and intermediate care facilities (NCHS, 1979).

The average cost of nursing home care per patient per month is now more than $1,500, and it has been estimated that as the population gets older, one out of four or one out of five Americans will have need for such nursing or personal care services (Comptroller General's Report, 1980).

An issue discussed earlier is the role of the long-term care institution as a mini-mental hospital. It has been estimated that two-thirds of all long-term care patients are taking psychotropic drugs (Moss & Halamandaris, 1977), that a majority of long-term care patients have significant psychiatric symptomatology (Eisdorfer & Stotsky, 1977), but that specialized mental health services are rarely provided in long-term care, partly because of lack of funding. Alternative therapeutic strategies are rarely employed since administrative staff and policymakers as well as clinicians usually do not know about such strategies.

The estimate that one-third of older Americans in nursing homes might be cared for on the outside is often quoted, although that figure is based on data from one study by a group of public health nurses and physicians in Florida (Bell, 1973). They estimated that one-third of the patients they had referred to nursing homes might be cared for in the community, given appropriate support. Unfortunately, "appropriate support" in the community is either not available or too expensive.

The current status of nursing home care is uncertain. Although nursing homes potentially represent a health resource, most are disconnected from the health care system or its educational bases. On the one hand, projections indicate that long-term care beds are likely to play an increasingly greater role (with the population of elderly and infirm persons growing), and on the other, the demand for community alternatives for institutional care is great. The difficulty lies in a failure to identify actual needs and develop appropriate resources. Nursing home policy is unfocused, and a continuation of the current preference for rhetoric over activity could result in an even more serious problem for long-term care in the next decade.

Programs to upgrade nursing home care have resulted in some improvement in facilities, with greater attention to safety standards and much talk about improvement of quality of life and patient care.

However, the paucity of professionals trained to work in such facilities, the low level of state payments under Medicaid, and the utilization of nursing homes as warehouses for the aged or as dumping grounds for those denied admission to state hospitals have resulted in an attitude of therapeutic nihilism. There are very few models of effective long-term care administration, although such models coupled with major health teaching agencies could be very valuable.

A biased position for or against any component of a caring system is unwarranted in the absence of research on the relative merits and liabilities of such components, e.g., nursing home, respite care, home health care, and so on. An appreciation of the value of home-based care and the development of good ties between the community and long-term care institutions is rare, despite its promise for more effective and cost-effective care.

Considerable attention has been given to the long-term care issue by Congress and the Federal Government (Comptroller General's Report, 1980) in part because costs are projected to escalate to $95 billion per year by 1990. The Federal Administration on Aging (AOA) has established a number of long-term care centers and has begun to focus on this area. It has been suggested that the 1980s will be the decade in which we finally come to grips with the long-term care issue. Training in long-term care settings is therefore an important component of any mental health curriculum.

9
Barriers to
Effective Long-term Care and
Alternative Strategies

Long-term care draws from more than one discipline to meet an older patient's multiple needs. Therefore, training in interdisciplinary health care settings is important to develop an individual's understanding of the problem of coordinated service delivery and to improve communication between collaborating health care professionals. Training experiences should also provide the professional with opportunities to conceptualize alternative health care strategies for the aged, and, where possible, to develop policies with economic, social and political scientists, as well as with information technologists, and perhaps even with corporate executives.

The growing population of older people confronts us with the need to develop a long-term care system that utilizes both hospital and community-based services for diagnosis, treatment, rehabilitation, and prevention (IOM, 1978). Unfortunately, the technological advances of modern medicine and health care are concentrated in the hospital, and this has resulted in an increased cost of hospital care and a dearth of services in the community.

While the life-enhancing potential of technology is clear, its disadvantages are less apparent. In medicine, technological advances are usually oriented toward a more sophisticated detection of disease and toward a small number of patients for whom a given technology provides appropriate treatment. The result is a focus upon those diseases for which we have technological solutions regardless of their overall impact on the human condition. Another disadvantage of burgeoning technology is the expensive period of overlap in which old and new techniques are used redundantly. The diagnosis of dementing illness is a case in point; skull X-rays, CT scans, isotope uptake studies, and cerebral blood flow studies are all used.

This is not an argument that technological advances are unnecessary. The point is that high technology is not the appropriate solution for all problems. It would be ludicrous, for example, to increase the mobility of a military unit by having every soldier drive his own tank. Similarly, it may be the wrong approach to focus on the hospital as the best place to provide care, and to continue to emphasize acute care with its high-technology strategies rather than the range of other services necessary for better health. Unfortunately, the number of hospital beds in the U.S. is in excess of our need, but in order to reduce the unit costs of expensive hospital operations, we continue to use these beds, and consequently drive health care costs higher.

High technology has come to equal high prestige, and both training and clinician reimbursement are bound tightly to technological philosophy. A physician earns more in an hour using diagnostic machines or performing surgery than by taking a careful history, doing a physical or psychiatric examination, identifying whether the patient understands the nature of the illness, or discussing the habits that produce or exacerbate illness. Since the physician is usually the patient's principle health advisor and determines the treatment required, the use of increased technology and an escalating cost of care result. However, the physician may be the victim as well as the perpetrator of this pattern of care.

Better hospitals have become synonymous with better equipment, drugs, and exotic procedures. Eisdorfer (1981) has emphasized that the hospital is an exhibition hall of American technophilia. Hospital staffs, hospital board members, governors, mayors, political leaders, and the public all show enthusiasm for building, but not for closing, hospitals, despite the potential for reducing general medical costs, tax benefits, and the availability of more funds for other, often more appropriate, health-related services.

Increased clinical technology and current patterns of third-party coverage may jeopardize rather than improve the future health care of the aged whose problems are chronic and involve functional incapacities, not just diseases and cures. It must be clearly understood that solutions to these problems are not solely medical but are political, social, and educational. A deep-rooted belief that hospitals and intensive-care institutions are the best means to provide care has made victims of the aging and aged, as well as of their families and caregivers.

The "medicalization" of the problems of the aged has had a number of unfortunate consequences. Medicare has elevated general health care and especially acute care above all other needs. Although the aged certainly have acute illnesses, the major health problems of older persons are chronic rather than acute. Appropriate treatment aims to maximize their capacity to care for themselves every day, and not just during short-term (acute) episodes of sickness. Increased functional dependence is both a social and a health problem but social benefits are not given the high priority of acute medical or hospital-based care.

Our failure to develop alternatives to nursing homes or alternatives within institutions has created a system that defeats rather than rewards family caregivers in the community. While families are shouldering the burdens of long-term care for older persons, our reimbursement system does not support them as a source of social and health care. Unfortunately, basing long-term care facilities upon the acute care model has made the term *long-term care* synonymous with nursing home institutions rather than with an effective and humane system of care for someone over a long period of time.

If technophilia exists in our country, it may also be accompanied by psychophobia—fear of dealing with the emotional and cognitive changes in people (Eisdorfer, 1981). Thus, as stated earlier, most patients in need of long-term care get little or no outpatient mental health care. The aged are given institutional care rather than access to a range of services that maximize functional independence and human dignity.

Innovative clinical approaches can alter or replace the hospital environment. The hospice movement has shown that a personalized pattern of socialization between staff, patient, and family can enhance the quality of the final weeks of life. In contrast, hospital-based technological solutions often make death sterile and expensive. Day hospitals, outpatient surgery, and alternative arrangements for childbirth are all being tried. Community- and housing-based health and social services, dental and health screening, and educational programs are being tested for their usefulness in promoting health among older community residents.

Funding levels competitive with those for institutions are needed for programs of health promotion and community-based management of disease. A medical and social triage system could be instituted to identify the array of needs of a specific patient, and then the appropriate combination of social and health services could be provided. This approach could reduce the need for institutionalization and help families maintain their relative in the community without exhausting financial and emotional resources. Such a health care program promotes the philosophy that the aged are an important asset to society, and that chronic illness is not a barrier to an important and meaningful social role.

This is not to deny that hospitals are an important component of the health care system. However, significant developments in the health care system are needed to effect a continuous program of health maintenance and a maximization of function. Follow-up care, including social, nutritional, home nursing, and other services, is necessary. Entitlements for certain medications would help ensure that the older patient follows medical advice and does not become the victim of a medication vs. lunch conflict.

Perhaps the single largest barrier to care is the disease-oriented nature of our training. Eisdorfer (1979) has traced the development of health care education and medicine along three vectors: the structural or organic approach, which emphasizes a variety of basic sciences, including anatomy, histology, and pathology, and such clinical arts as surgery; the humoral approach, which is now institutionalized as biochemistry, pharmacology, and the practice of internal medicine; and the behavioral approach, for the diagnosis and management of behaviors that were once the sign of demonic possession and were not labeled as psychiatric disorders, e.g., depression, bad habits (smoking, overeating), chronic pain, and such interpersonal difficulties as marital conflict.

Although these three approaches overlap somewhat, the basic and clinical education of health care professionals follows these vectors. Society has clearly indicated its preference.

> The organ-oriented physician provides services linked to high technology and gains the most fruit with the least time. This is not a criticism of high surgical fees, which may be justified by long training, delay of gratification and short productive life span as well as technical skills (like football or basketball stars). Rather it is to point out that the training of medical students, nurses and a variety of health professionals, as well as the structure of the hospitals supported by our society, have made this approach the most lucrative if not powerful and prestigious.
>
> The humoralist-physician functions with more or less good humor in the same setting, but also with a foot outside the high technology system. Yet he/she, like the organicist, has been trained to deal with the exotic component and given intensive experience in brief interludes with patients who are usually grouped to show similar biochemical problems and receive similar pharmacologic therapy, e.g., the diabetes clinic, the arthritis clinic, or the hypertension clinic.
>
> The behavioralist behaves in the strangest fashion of all. Some recognize that behavior relates to the existence of the body but because of poor training, or a narrow belief system, or because some of the non-medical, non-nursing professionals don't have the body included in their legal franchise, they choose to ignore it entirely. Others are so beset with the new humoral knowledge finally emerging from studies of the central and autonomic nervous system and relations to the immune system, that the patients' feelings, beliefs, families and ecosystems play little or no part in their perception and treatment of behavior [Eisdorfer, 1979].

Another approach is needed to provide quality care for those who are old today and all of us who will be old tomorrow. Neither the structural, the humoral, nor the behavioral approach is valid alone, since none can serve all the patient's needs. A complex system of integrated care is required to promote health and happiness.

Unless our training addresses the changing needs of the patients within their changing ecosystems, we will continue to chase our own tails in a spiral of increasing costs and more specialized services which fractionate rather than integrate the care of the aged and everyone else.

Appendix:
Program Evaluation Forms

1. END-OF ROTATION REPORT

Date of this Report_____

Service_____

Service Chief _____

Name of Trainee _____

Please complete the following report and return to _____

_____ at your earliest convenience. This report is reviewed

by the Evaluation Committee and is considered in regard to letters

of recommendation from the department in later years. This report

will be summarized and discussed with the individual by the faculty

advisor.

COMPLETION OF THIS FORM IS NOT NECESSARY IF YOU HAVE PERSONALLY

SUBMITTED QUARTERLY REPORTS ON THIS TRAINEE. HOWEVER, PLEASE

RETURN THIS FORM FOR OUR RECORDS.

Please comment on those of the following items of which you have
knowledge or an opinion:

Professional demeanor and appearance:

Ability to relate to peers and other professionals while on your
service:

What are this individual's strong points?

In what areas does this individual need to acquire additional skill
or knowledge?

Other problem areas of which you are aware:

109

2. QUARTERLY SUPERVISOR'S REPORT FOR THE PERIOD _____

Supervisor _____ Service _____

Name of Trainee_____

Please complete the following report and return to _____

at your earliest convenience. We hope that you will share the infor-

mation contained in this report with your supervisee. This report

becomes a part of the trainee's departmental file. It is reviewed by

the Postdoctoral Evaluation Committee and is considered in regard to

letters of recommendation from the department in later years.

How many times have you supervised this individual?

How would you rate this person's overall professional expertise and
performance on a scale of 1 to 10 (10 being superior)?

What are this person's strong points?

In what areas does this person need to acquire additional skill or
knowledge?

Would you feel comfortable referring a patient to this individual
for psychiatric evaluation or treatment?

Please comment on those of the following items of which you have
knowledge or an opinion:

Professional demeanor and appearance:

Ability to relate to peers and other professionals:

Ability to relate effectively to patients and to spouse and family
of patients:

Flexibility and open-mindedness of approach:

Intellectual curiosity:

110

Interest and ability as a teacher:

Diagnostic and clinical judgment:

Knowledge of psychodynamics:

Knowledge of pharmacotherapeutics:

Ability to relate general medical and/or psychological knowledge to psychiatric knowledge:

Apparent knowledge of current psychiatric literature:

Apparent knowledge of psychotherapy:

Thoroughness of workups:

Promptness of workups:

Day-to-day handling of case management (where applicable):

Conscientiousness about completing paper work including letters to referring doctors, etc.:

3. QUARTERLY RESEARCH REPORT

Supervisory Report on _____ Supervisor: _____

Period of Supervision: _____, 198_ Elective: RESEARCH

Please complete the following report and return to_____

_____

What is your overall appraisal of this trainee as a potential
researcher?

Poor   _____   Comments:

Fair   _____

Satisfactory _____

Good   _____

Very Good   _____

Superior   _____

_____

Please evaluate the following items and add your comments:

_____

Poor   _____   Ability to formulate a research problem;
                         originality:
Fair   _____

Satisfactory _____

Good   _____

Very Good   _____

Superior   _____

_____

Poor   _____   Initiative and scholarly interest, including
                         knowledge of relevant literature in the
Fair   _____   field:

Satisfactory _____

Good   _____

Very Good   _____

Superior   _____

_____

Poor	_____	Knowledge of statistics and experimental design:
Fair	_____	
Satisfactory	_____	
Good	_____	
Very Good	_____	
Superior	_____	

Poor	_____	Ability to perform relevant experimental techniques for this type of research, for example, manipulative, electronics, or apparatus skills:
Fair	_____	
Satisfactory	_____	
Good	_____	
Very Good	_____	
Superior	_____	

Poor	_____	Perserverance in completing the project:
Fair	_____	
Satisfactory	_____	
Good	_____	
Very Good	_____	
Superior	_____	

Poor	_____	Degree of independence from supervisor; ability to work out most of problem alone, potential to be an independent researcher:
Fair	_____	
Satisfactory	_____	
Good	_____	
Very Good	_____	
Superior	_____	

Poor   _____   <u>Flexibility; ability to take advice and
                              criticism, abandoning a point of view if
Fair   _____   it proves untenable:</u>

Satisfactory   _____

Good   _____

Very Good   _____

Superior   _____

Poor   _____   <u>Administration; Ability to write up
                              reports, get analysis and other paperwork
Fair   _____   completed:</u>

Satisfactory   _____

Good   _____

Very Good   _____

Superior   _____

114

4. DIDACTIC EVALUATION

Good teaching and good teachers are maintained by feedback; poor
teaching is improved by it. Your ratings of and comments about the
didactic program thus far are vital. Please complete the question-
naire frankly and return it at your earliest convenience. Circle
the appropriate numbers: 1 to indicate lowest ratings and 7 the
highest.

NOTE: Your comments will greatly help the evaluation procedure and
       are encouraged. Ratings of 1 or 7 especially should be
       accompanied by comments.

Didactic/Seminar_____ Coordinator or
                                  Primary Teacher_____

Year of training: 1 2   Date(Qtr.)_____

A. Global rating of value and interest of this   1 2 3 4 5 6 7
    course for you.

    Comments:

B. Style and Structure

    1. Adequate preparation of lecture(s).   1 2 3 4 5 6 7

        Comments:

    2. Adequate presentation of material
        (clarity, stimulation, etc.).   1 2 3 4 5 6 7

        Comments:

C. Content

    1. Was course useful and relevant to your
        current needs?   1 2 3 4 5 6 7

        Comments:

    2. Adequate breadth of coverage.   1 2 3 4 5 6 7

        Comments:

    3. Adequate depth of coverage.   1 2 3 4 5 6 7

        Comments:

    4. Adequate readings.   1 2 3 4 5 6 7

        Comments:

    5. Proper sequence in your program.   1 2 3 4 5 6 7

        Comments:

115

D. Attendance is an indicator of course quality. If this course was a series, estimate your attendance rate.

E. What was good about this course/lecture?

F. In what ways could this course/lecture be improved?

Additional comments and/or suggestions:

116

BIBLIOGRAPHY

Bibliography

Akpom, C. A., & Mayer, S. A survey of geriatric education in U.S. medical schools. *Journal of Medical Education*, 1978, *53*, 66–68.

Bell, W. G. Community care for the elderly: An alternative to institutionalization. *Gerontologist*, 1973, *13*, 349–354.

Bernstein, I., Bohrnstedt, G. W., & Borgatta, E. F. External validity and evaluation research. Codification of problems. *Sociological Methods and Research*, 1975, *4*, 101–128.

Blazer, D., & Williams, C. D. Epidemiology of dysphoria and depression in an elderly population. *American Journal of Psychiatry*, 1980, *137*, 439–444.

Blenkner, M. Environmental change and the aging individual. *Gerontologist*, 1967, 7, 101–105.

Blumenthal, M. O., Davie, J. W., & Morycz, R. K. Developing a curriculum in psychogeriatrics. *American Journal of Psychiatry*, 1979, *136*, 1157–1161.

Bremer, F. A social psychiatric investigation of a small community in northern Norway. *Acta Psychiatrica Neurologica Scandinavica*, 1951, *62* (Supplement 1).

Brocklehurst, J. C. (ed.), *Textbook of geriatric medicine and gerontology*. Edinburgh: Churchill Livingstone, 1973.

Brody, S. J. Health policy. *Generations*, 1981, *6*, 1–5.

Brody, S. J., Poulshock, S. W., & Masciocchi, C. F. The family caring unit: A major consideration in the long-term support system. *Gerontologist*, 1978, *18*, 558–559.

Brotman, H. B. Every ninth American. In *Developments in aging*. U.S. Special Committee on Aging, 1980.

Busse, E. W., Dovenmuehle, R. H., & Brown, R. G. Psychoneurotic reactions of the aged. *Geriatrics*, 1960, *15*, 97–105.

Busse, E. W., & Pfeiffer, E. Functional psychiatric disorders in old age. In E. W. Busse & E. Pfeiffer (Eds.), *Behavior and adaptation in late life*. Boston: Little, Brown, 1975.

Butler, R. N. Psychiatry and the elderly: An overview. *American Journal of Psychiatry*, 1975, *132*, 893–900.

Butler, R. N. Geriatrics and internal medicine. *Annals of Internal Medicine*, 1979, *91*, 903–908.

Cain, G. *Evaluation and Experiment*. New York: Academic Press, 1975.

Campbell, D. T., & Stanley, J. C. *Experimental and quasi-experimental designs for research*. Chicago: Rand McNally, 1966.

Cantor, M., & Mayer M. *Health crisis for older New Yorkers. Facts for action series*. New York: Office for the Aging, 1972.

Cohen, D., & Wu, S. Language and cognition during aging. In C. Eisdorfer & B. Starr (Eds.), *Annual review of geriatrics and gerontology*. New York: Springer, 1980.

Cohen, G. D. Mental health services and the elderly: needs and options. *American Journal of Psychiatry*, 1976, *133*, 65–68.

Comptroller General's Report to the Congress. *Entering a nursing home— costly implications for Medicaid and the elderly*. Washington, D.C.: General Accounting Office, PAD-80-12, 1980.

Cyrus-Lutz, C., & Gaitz, C. M. Psychiatrists' attitudes toward the aged and aging. *Gerontologist*, 1972, *12*, 163–167.

Dans, P. E., & Kerr, M. Gerontology and geriatrics in medical education. *New England Journal of Medicine*, 1979, *300*, 228–232.

Eisdorfer, C. Evaluation of the quality of psychiatric care for the aged. *American Journal of Psychiatry*, 1977, *134*, 315–317.

Eisdorfer, C. Psychophysiologic and cognitive studies in the aged. In G. Usdin & C. J. Hofling (Eds.), *Aging: The process and the people*. New York: Brunner-Mazel, 1978.

Eisdorfer, C. The future of aging and the training of health care professionals. The Joseph T. Freeman lecture delivered at the Gerontological Society Annual Meeting, Washington, D.C., 1979.

Eisdorfer, C. Paranoia and schizophrenic disorders in late life. In E. W. Busse & D. G. Blazer (Eds.), *Handbook of geriatric psychiatry*. New York: Van Nostrand Reinhold, 1980.

Eisdorfer, C. Care of the aged: the barriers of traditions. *Annals of Internal Medicine*, 1981, *94*, 256–260.

Eisdorfer, C., & Basen M. Drug misuse by the elderly. In R. Dupont, A. Goldstein, & J. O'Donnell (Eds.), *Handbook on drug abuse*. Washington, D.C.: NIDA, USDHEW and Office of Drug Abuse Policy, Executive Office of the President, 1979.

Eisdorfer, C., & Cohen, D. The cognitively impaired elderly: Differential diagnosis. In M. Storandt, I. Seigler, & M. F. Elias (Eds.), *The clinical psychology of aging*. New York: Plenum, 1978.

Eisdorfer, C., & Cohen, D. Diagnostic criteria for primary neuronal degeneration of the Alzheimer's type. *Journal of Family Practice,* 1980, *11,* 553–557.

Eisdorfer, C., Cohen, D., & Preston, C. Behavioral and psychological therapies for dementing illness. In N. Miller & G. D. Cohen (Eds.), *The clinical aspects of Alzheimer's disease and senile dementia.* New York: Raven Press, 1981.

Eisdorfer, C., & Stotsky, B. A. Intervention, treatment, and rehabilitation of psychiatric disorders. In J. E. Birren & K. W. Schaie (Eds.), *Handbook of the psychology of aging.* New York: Van Nostrand Reinhold, 1977.

Ferguson Anderson, W. *Practical management of the elderly.* Oxford: Blackwell Scientific Publications, 1971.

Freeman, J. T. A survey of geriatric education: catalogues of United States medical schools. *Journal of the American Geriatric Society,* 1971, *19,* 746–762.

Gibson, R. M., & Fisher, C. R. Age differences in health care spending, Fiscal Year 1977. HCFA Health Note, December 1978.

Gibson, R. M., Mueller, M. S., & Fisher, C. R. Age difference in health care spending, fiscal year 1976. *Social Security Bulletin,* 1977, *40,* 3–14.

Goldman, R. Geriatrics as a specialty—Problems and prospects. *Gerontologist,* 1974, *14,* 468–471.

Gruenberg, D. Epidemiology of senile dementia. In R. Katzman, R. Terry, & K. Bick (Eds.), *Alzheimer's disease, senile dementia, and related disorders.* New York: Raven Press, 1978.

Gurland, B. J. The comparative frequency of depression in various adult age groups. *Journal of Gerontology,* 1976, *31,* 283–292.

Gurland, B., Dean, L., Cross, P., & Golden, R. The epidemiology of depression and dementia in the elderly: The use of multiple indicators of these conditions. In J. O. Cole & J. E. Barrett (Eds.), *Psychopathology in the aged.* New York: Raven Press, 1980.

Health Care Financing Administration. Long-term care: background and future directions. HCFA 81–20047, 1981.

Hickey, T., Rakowski, W., Hultsch, D. F. Attitudes toward aging as a function of in-service training and practitioner age. *Journal of Gerontology,* 1976, *31,* 681–686.

Holtzman, J., Beck, J. D., Hodgetts, P. G., Coggan, P. G., & Ryan, N. Geriatrics program for medical students. II: Impact of two educational experiences on student attitudes. *Journal of the American Geriatric Society,* 1978, *26,* 355–359.

Institute of Medicine. *Aging and medical education*. Washington, D. C.: National Academy of Sciences, 1978.

Jarvik, L. F., Eisdorfer, C., & Blum, J. E. (Eds.). *Intellectual functioning in adults*. New York: Springer, 1973.

Kahana, E., & Coe, R. M. Self and staff conceptions of institutionalized aged. *Gerontologist*, 1969, 9, 264–267.

Kane, R. L., Solomon, D. H., Beck, J. C., Keeler, E., & Kane, R. A. *Geriatrics in the United States: Manpower projections and training considerations*. Santa Monica, Calif.: Rand, R-2543-HJK, 1980.

Katzman, R., & Karasu, T. B. Differential diagnosis of dementia. In W. S. Fields (Ed.), *Neurological and sensory disorders in the elderly*. New York: Grune & Stratton, 1975.

Kay, D. W. K. The epidemiology of brain deficit in the aged: Problems in patient identification. In C. Eisdorfer & R. O. Friedel (Eds.), *The cognitively and emotionally impaired aged*. Chicago: Yearbook Medical Publications, 1977.

Kay, D. W. K., Beamish, P., & Roth, M. Old age mental disorders in Newcastle-upon-Tyne. Part I. A study of prevalence. *British Journal of Psychiatry*, 1964, *110*, 146–158.

Kidd, C. B. Misplacement of the elderly in hospital. A study of patients admitted to geriatric and mental hospitals. *British Medical Journal*, 1962, *5318*, 1491–1495.

Kilty, K. M. & Feld, A. Attitudes toward aging and towards the needs of older people. *Journal of Gerontology*, 1976, *31*, 586–594.

Kogan, N. Attitudes toward old people: the development of a scale and an examination of correlates. *Journal of Abnormal Social Psychology*, 1961, *62*, 44–54.

Kosberg, J. I., Cohen, S. Z. & Mendlovitz, A. Comparison of supervisors' attitudes in a home for the aged. *Gerontologist*, 1972, *12*, 241–245.

Kovar, M. G. Elderly people: The population 65 years and over. In *Health, United States, 1976–1977*. Washington, D. C.: Department of Health, Education, and Welfare, DHEW Publication No. (HRA) 77–1232, 1977.

Kramer, M. The rising pandemic of mental disorders and associated chronic diseases and disabilities. *Acta Psychiatrica Scandinavica*, 1980, Suppl. 285, 62, 383–396.

Kramer, M., Taube, C. A., & Redick, R. W. Patterns of use of psychiatric facilities by the aged: Past, present, and future. In C. Eisdorfer, & M. P. Lawton (Eds.), *The psychology of adult development and aging*. Washington, D. C.: American Psychological Association, 1973.

Labouvie-Vief, G. Adaptive dimensions of adult cognition. In N. Datan & N. Lohman (Eds.). *Transitions of aging*. New York: Academic Press, 1980.

Leaf, A. Sounding board. Medicine and the aged. *New England Journal of Medicine*, 1977, *297*, 887–890.

Libow, L. S. Pseudo-senility: acute and reversible organic brain syndromes. *Journal of the American Geriatric Society*, 1973, *21*, 112–120.

Libow, L. S. A geriatric medical residency program. A four-year experience. *Annals of Internal Medicine*, 1976, *85*, 641–647.

Lowenthal, M. J., & Berkman, P. L. *Aging and mental disorder in San Francisco. A social psychiatric study*. San Francisco: Jossey-Bass, 1967.

Miller, D. B., Lowenstein, R., & Winston, R. Physicians' attitudes toward the ill aged and nursing homes. *Journal of the American Geriatric Society*, 1976, *24*, 498–505.

Moss, F. E., & Halamandaris, V. J. *Too old too sick too bad*. Germantown, Md.: Aspen, 1977.

National Center for Health Statistics. *The national nursing home survey: 1977 summary for the United States*. Vital and Health Statistics Series 13, No. 43. DHEW Publication No. (PHS) 79-1794, 1979.

Noelker, L., & Harel, Z. Predictors of well-being and survival among institutionalized aged. *Gerontologist*, 1978, *18*, 562–567.

Panneton, P. E., & Wesolowski, E. F. Current and future needs in geriatric education. *Public Health Reports*, 1979, *94*, 73–79.

Perry, B. C. Proposed evaluation design for University of Washington Medical School geriatrics curriculum. Seattle, 1980. Mimeographed.

Poe, W. D. Letter: Education in geriatrics. *Journal of Medical Education*, 1975, *50*, 1002–1003.

Reichel, W. (Ed.). Proceedings of the American Geriatric Society conferences on geriatric education. *Journal of the American Geriatric Society*, 1977, *25*, 481–513.

Riedel, R. L., & Riedel, D. C. *Practice and performance: An assessment of ambulatory care*. Ann Arbor, Mich.: Health Administration Press, 1979.

Rodstein, M. A model curriculum for an elective course in geriatrics. *Gerontologist*, 1973, *12*, 231–235.

Rosencrantz, H. A., & McNevin, T. E. A factor analysis of attitudes toward the aged. *Gerontologist*, 1969, *9*, 55–59.

Rossman, I. J. (Ed.). *Clinical geriatrics*. Philadelphia: J. B. Lippincott, 1971.

Schaie, K. W. Toward a stage theory of adult cognitive development. *International Journal of Aging & Human Development*, 1977-8, *8*, 129–138.

Schuckit, M. A. Geriatric alcoholism and drug abuse. *Gerontologist*, 1977, *17*, 168–174. (a)

Schuckit, M. A. The high rate of psychiatric disorders in elderly cardiac patients. *Angiology*, 1977, *28*, 235–247. (b)

Schuckit, M. A., Miller, P. L., & Hahlbohm, D. Unrecognized psychiatric illness in elderly medical-surgical patients. *Journal of Gerontology*, 1975, *30*, 655–660.

Shortell, S. M., & Richardson, W. C. *Health program evaluation*. St. Louis: C. V. Mosby, 1978.

Somers, A. R. Geriatric care in the United Kingdom: an American perspective. *Annals of Internal Medicine*, 1976, *84*, 466–476.

Somers, H. M., & Somers, A. R. *Medicare and the hospitals*. Washington, D. C.: Brookings Institution, 1967.

Stevens, R. Geriatric medicine in historical perspective: the pros and cons of geriatric medicine as a specialty. Working Paper #1, Tulane Studies in Health Policy, 1977. Mimeographed.

Tomlinson, B. E., Blessed, G., & Roth, M. Observations on the brains of demented old people. *Journal of the Neurological Sciences*, 1970, *11*, 205–242.

Tuckman, J., & Lorge, I. Attitudes toward old people. *Journal of Social Psychology*, 1953, *37*, 249–260.

Weinberger, L. E., & Milham, J. A multi-dimensional, multiple method analysis of attitudes toward the elderly. *Journal of Gerontology*, 1975, *30*, 343–348.

Weiss, C. H. *Evaluation research: Methods of assessing program effectiveness*. Englewood Cliffs, N.J.: Prentice-Hall, 1972.

Wells, C. E. *Dementia* (2nd ed.). Philadelphia: Davis Co., 1977.

Wells, C. E. Pseudodementia. *American Journal of Psychiatry*, 1979, *136*, 895–900.

Wolk, R. L., & Wolk, R. B. Professional workers' attitudes toward the aged. *Journal of the American Geriatric Society*, 1971, *19*, 624–639.

Wright, I. S. Geriatrics—the challenges of the seventies: rethinking and retooling for the future. *Journal of the American Geriatric Society*, 1971, *19*, 737–745.

Index

Index

Acute Care Unit, year 1 rotation in, 22–25
Acute inpatient care skills, 19
Administration on Aging (AOA), 91, 99
Advanced Clinician track, 16, 26
Aged
  complex nature of illnesses, 6
  demography of, 3, 87–88
  expectation of sickness in, 92–93
  health care utilization by, 3, 81–82
  health strategies for, 65–66
  life expectancy of, 85
  in nursing homes, 81–82
  personality and intellectual changes in, 37, 83–84
  population in need of mental health services, 3, 85
Aging, normal, 35, 36–38
  theories of, 37–38
Aging and geriatric psychiatry seminar, 27
Alcoholism, 5, 10, 83, 84, 93
  manifestation and management of, 48–49
Alzheimer's disease, 19–20, 43, 84
Antianxiety drugs, 52
Antidepressant drugs, 52
Antimanic drugs, 52
Antipsychotic drugs, 52
Anxiety disorders, manifestation and management of, 47
Attending teaching rounds, 27

Behavioral assessment of psychopathology, 39–41
Behavioral management, as strategy, 53–54
Biological theories of aging, 37

Chronic Care Unit, year 1 rotation in, 22–25
Chronic illness statistics, 87
Chronic inpatient care skills, 19–20
Classroom training, 26–33
Clinical care program
  attitudes, 17
  classroom and conference training, 26–33
  knowledge, 17–18
  rotation for clinical practice specialty and academically oriented professionals, 22–26
  skills, 16–17
  training sites and their skill opportunities, 18–22
  two-year, 16–33
  see also Curriculum on mental health and aging
Clinical psychology gerontologists, 8, 15, 20
Clinical Research and Teaching track, 16, 22, 26
Clinical tests for dementing illness, 43–44
Clinical training sites, 18–22
Cognitive-acting drugs, 52–53